P9-DWQ-180

12,000 CANARIES CAN'T BE WRONG

What's making us sick,
and what you can do about it

John Molot, M.D.

ECW Press

Copyright © John Molot, 2014

Published by ECW Press
2120 Queen Street East, Suite 200
Toronto, Ontario, Canada M4E 1E2
416-694-3348 / info@ecwpress.com

LIBRARY AND ARCHIVES CANADA CATALOGING IN PUBLICATION

Molot, John, 1946–, author
12,000 canaries can't be wrong : what's making us sick
and what you can do about it / John Molot, M.D.

Previously published: 12,000 canaries can't be wrong : what's making you
sick and what you can do / Dr. John Molot. — Toronto : EnviroHealth Publications, 2013.

ISBN: 978-1-77041-133-3 (BOUND)
Also issued as: 978-1-77090-563-4 (EPUB); 978-1-77090-562-7 (PDF)

1. Environmental health. 2. Environmentally induced diseases.

I. Title. II. Title: Twelve thousand canaries can't be wrong. III. Title: What's making
us sick and what you can do about it. IV. Title: What's making you sick and what you can do.

RA566.M65 2014   616.9'8   C2014-901295-0   C2014-901296-9

Cover design: Rachel Ironstone
Cover image: canary: tunart / iStock
Typesetting and production: Lynn Gammie
Printing: Friesens 1 2 3 4 5

ECW Press acknowledges the financial support of the Government of Canada through the Canada Book Fund for our publishing activities, and the contribution of the Government of Ontario through the Ontario Book Publishing Tax Credit and the Ontario Media Development Corporation.

PRINTED AND BOUND IN CANADA

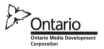
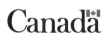

DEDICATION

To my parents, Dave and Lotte, for being who they were, and for never allowing me to give up;

To Helen and Lewis, my siblings and my best friends;

To my children: Noah and Josh, for being appreciative and encouraging and making me proud; and Samantha, for enabling me to see the world through a different and better lens;

To my brother Morris, whose death initiated my journey towards writing this book.

CONTENTS

Part III | Environmental Illness

Part IV | The Environmental Link with Chronic Illness

Part V | What You Can Do

Part VI | The Environment of Medicine

ACKNOWLEDGEMENTS

Thank you to all my patients, for allowing me into their lives and letting me learn from their experiences;

to the many thousands of dedicated scientists whose published work supplied the wealth of data in this book, for providing the data to finally and powerfully respond to the cynicism and ignorance of those who still erroneously and harmfully advocate that the science upholding the practice of environmental medicine is junk;

to Mark Lazarovitz, for his continuous support and encouragement to write this book;

to David Wineberg, who coaxed and coached and taught me more English in one year than all my teachers in high school;

to Arnold Gosewich, for his honesty and expertise;

to Robby, Kevin, and Annie Shore, for their ideas, examples, and suggestions;

to those who worked on the original edition: Leon Mintz, for his graphic support, Gillian Watts, for her copy editing and index, Angel Guerra, for the book design, and Andris Pone, for naming this book;

to Arlene Anthony, Sam and Esther Cukierman, Jean Golden, Jaimini Randev, Henry Molot, Lewis Molot, Lynn Marshall, Jayne Hobbs, Rickey Held, and Vincent Chetcuti, for their careful reading and thoughtful suggestions;

to Marie-Andree Doyon, my admin, and Carol Ciasnocha, my nurse, for their unfailing, enduring partnerships with me, for their participation in the care and support of thousands of patients seen together over the past 30 years, and for their wisdom and friendship;

and most of all to my wife, Debra Aronson, for listening to all my rants, for helping to transform them into this book, and especially for making it comprehensible for everyone else; for her perseverance and inspiration; for her enduring labour, without which this project would have failed; for all the magical, muted, rejuvenating appearances of bowls of fruit and vegetables; for her unwavering belief in me; and for her smile.

INTRODUCTION

In 1986, technology replaced the old tradition of using canaries to detect carbon monoxide in coal mines. Miners would take them underground because the canary is particularly sensitive to the gas, and any sign of distress from the canary was a clear signal warning that environmental conditions in the mine were unsafe and that the miners should be evacuated.

Over the past 30 years I have assessed and followed more than 12,000 patients with chronic medical conditions linked to the environment. Consider them human canaries warning that our environment is unsafe even if the rest of us can't detect it. Many of these people have distressing symptoms that they attribute to multiple common chemical exposures at levels that the rest of us tolerate. This condition is called multiple chemical sensitivities.

This experience also provided me with the opportunity to eventually see a pattern of illness that defied explanation. My curiosity and fascination with what I have observed in my medical practice has driven me to scrutinize the literature in cell biology, toxicology, pharmacology, epidemiology, and environmental health. However, most doctors have refused to accept the possibility that the pattern of illness in these patients could be real, that exposures to low levels of chemicals that we all seem to be tolerating could be making people sick. Instead, they told these patients that the symptoms were "in their heads." This denial, which stigmatized and discriminated against my patients, motivated me to persevere, to try to understand, to consolidate, and to remain up-to-date with the increasingly relentless flow of new information regarding the impact of pollution exposure on human biology.

The evidence now validates and explains the existence of environmentally related conditions. The existence of multiple chemical sensitivities, myalgic encephalomyelitis/chronic fatigue syndrome, fibromyalgia, and sick building syndrome can no longer be refuted. Not only that, the human canaries were right. These conditions turn out to be just the tip of a giant iceberg.

Humanity is facing a huge challenge. In *12,000 Canaries Can't Be Wrong: What's Making Us Sick, and What You Can Do About It*, you will read about how pollution evolution is pushing us along a continuum that is leading to the emergence of more and more cases of chronic disease, starting even in early childhood. But this book is not intended to be apocalyptic. You will gain an understanding of the mechanisms behind it all and be better informed about what you can do about it.

Environmental medicine has been discredited or ignored by critics who claim a lack of scientific evidence. That opinion is no longer justified. The concepts in this book are based on information found in more than 2,000 articles from the medical literature published in the peer-reviewed journals of many health and biology disciplines. All the studies can be found in the database of the U.S. National Library of Medicine.

For those who wish to see just how strong the evidence is, there is a sister version of this book available on JohnMolot.com. *12,000 Canaries Can't Be Wrong: Establishing the New Era of Environmental Medicine* contains more than 2,000 references. Every scientific statement is supported, sometimes with many citations. It demonstrates how robust the science now is in support of the concepts of environmental medicine.

Successful chronic disease prevention and management is predicated on individualized person-centred care and empowerment. *12,000 Canaries Can't Be Wrong* will provide you with the information required to make informed decisions to protect yourself and your family, including your future children and grandchildren. You can experience a better quality of health for a longer period of time.

— John Molot, M.D. CCFP FCFP

PART I

ENVIRONMENTAL MEDICINE

NAME_____ AGE_____
ADDRESS_____ DATE_____

☐ LABEL
REFILL 0 1 2 3 4 5   _____
                            (SIGNATURE)

CHAPTER 1

AN END AND A BEGINNING

Life is what happens while you're busy making other plans.
— Allen Saunders

I was 20 years old when I entered medical school. I was young and immature but willing to work hard and learn. It was the 1960s. I refused to wear a tie and grew my hair long enough to be told to wear a nurse's cap in surgery. Life was easy; my youthful rebellion was frivolous.

I was partway through my fourth-year obstetrics rotation when my brother Morris died. I was watching new lives being born into this world while my 16-year-old brother lay paralyzed on the living room couch at home, dying of brain cancer. On September 22, 1970, I came home from the hospital to find that he had stopped breathing. I listened to Morris's chest for the heartbeat that was no longer there and told my father, standing beside me, that the moment he was dreading had arrived. Then I went into the kitchen to break the news to my mother. I had just come home from assisting women in the birth of their children, and now I had to tell my own mother that Morris, the baby of our family, was dead. Not surprised but surprisingly stunned, I then went across the street to ask our neighbour, a dermatologist and one of my teachers at the university, to come to our home to officially pronounce my brother dead and help initiate the necessary processes and paperwork. At first he declined because he didn't know what to do.

Until that year the expectations that I had for myself as a physician were conventional, and encouraged by others. I was not going to be "just" a GP. After spending six weeks working with and being inspired by Dr. Wilbert Keon, a world-famous cardiovascular surgeon, I had chosen cardiology as my specialty, and I was accepted into the internal medicine residency training program at the Montreal General Hospital. But the person who had made the decision to follow that path had passed away with Morris on the living room sofa. Before I had completed my first year in Montreal, I realized that I was no longer suited for learning in that kind of environment. I was not the kind of person who could look at medicine from that same, conventional perspective anymore. I had been given too strong a dose of humility — even bitterness — that prevented me from feeling the enjoyment that my peers seemed to feel. I felt alienated as they displayed their knowledge by citing authors and journals that provided all the allegedly right solutions for treatment of the sick.

I needed to get away, to take some time off to decide what kind of doctor I wanted to be. I had become a 26-year-old licensed physician, armed with the latest medical education and understanding of how the human animal functioned. I had been taught to diagnose, to find the patient's pathology in some organ system, or otherwise to attribute what I could not explain to their alleged emotional flaws, and I was well trained to treat them accordingly. But being personally exposed to such an unfair death and witnessing the raw emotional pain that I observed in my parents had left me bewildered and cynical. Although consciously unaware of it, I had become bitter and contemptuous of the affectations of my superiors, the organ specialists. My brother died and they were no help. All I knew was that I needed to learn more, perhaps to see the human organism through a different lens. I spent many months catching up on the humanities, reading philosophy under a tree in the summertime, devouring novels, practising yoga and meditation, travelling in Europe, driving a tractor on a kibbutz in Israel, and finally returning home to start a general practice in a community clinic setting.

In the next few years I also became a husband and father. I nurtured a thriving practice as a family doctor in the city of Ottawa. Years later I remember sitting on top of a cliff on an island near Vancouver Island, watching the birds soar above the ocean below me, thinking how lucky I was to have a lovely family, two healthy, happy little boys, an interesting and wonderful profession, and a third child on the way. Life seemed rich and gratifying until four weeks later, when my daughter was born with severe hydrocephaly and a future life already impacted by significant brain damage.

Hydrocephaly is a condition in which an abnormal accumulation of fluid in the brain causes enlargement of the skull and compression of the brain. The neurosurgeon put in a shunt and fixed the hydrocephaly, but he couldn't repair her damaged brain. Anxious and confused, I wondered again how something like this could happen. Flooding back came those feelings of helplessness, bitterness, anger, and contempt for those who claimed to know the condition and to understand what had just happened to my family and me.

This was the start of my journey into the world of chronic illness. I have lived it on behalf of my daughter, because she didn't just enter our world — she obliged her family to live in and experience hers. I have learned to see what our world looks like under the burden of severe visual deficit, reduced physical strength and balance, and cognitive impairment. Unbeknownst to her, people stare because she looks different, but her life is enhanced by innocence, joy, a wonderful sense of humour, great communication skills, and sincere love for all the people in her orbit. Her view is unencumbered by her almost total dependence on others for care and protection, and she adds to the lives of those who allow her entry into their personal sphere.

How lucky she is not to fear for her future. Unfortunately, the government and its existing social safety network don't either. Well before I ever heard about the biopsychosocial model of health and disease I learned about the emotional and social impact of chronic illness, not as a physician learning from academia but as a father experiencing life. My mentor during this time was my mother. I remember telling her, after the birth of my daughter, how I now had a taste of her experience with my brother's illness. Her response was that it was the same, except for the outcome. I couldn't understand. Like any parent, I cannot fathom the concept of the death of my child. Thirty years after Morris died, when my daughter was 10 years old, my mother told me that eventually some healing had taken place for her, but she wondered how anyone can ever heal from the ongoing experience of parenting a damaged living child for the rest of their life.

This book is the outcome of my own experiences as a brother and a son, as a father, and as a student. I was traumatized enough by life's experiences to question the dogma of my medical school training. As a physician I was frustrated by awareness of my inability to be much help to those with chronic illness, except to provide pharmacological symptomatic Band-Aids. It is also the result of the fortunate twist of fate of being introduced, 30 years ago, to the fledgling concepts of environmental medicine and somehow having the inner strength or the anger to reject the criticism for accepting them. The rest of this book contains information from an environmental perspective that I hope will provide new and different insights on how to achieve and maintain a better quality of life for as long as possible, and perhaps to prevent the development of chronic illness in our children, even those as yet unborn.

New Concepts

To raise new questions, new possibilities, to regard old problems from a new angle, requires creative imagination and marks real advance in science.

— Albert Einstein

Most of us do not think about our inevitable demise unless its imminence becomes suddenly apparent in the doctor's office. We are never ready for that. None of us plans to die racked with cancerous pain and dependent on opium derivatives, or drowning in our own fluids because of a neuro-degenerative disorder, or suddenly while shovelling the driveway before our kids have even finished with school, or slowly, after years of living in a nursing home, confused by the apparent strangers who keep calling us Mom or Dad. However it ends, our life is a journey to that point, and how we get there depends on our gene pool, our lifestyle, the environment we live in, and luck. Unfortunately, in order to live as long as we can in good health, all we can manipulate is our lifestyle and environment. For many of us it is already too late because we have developed a chronic illness and life has been permanently and negatively altered.

The problem with chronic illness is that it's chronic. It has an impact on our physical well-being, our emotional perspective on quality of life, and the lives of those near and dear. We can manipulate it, mask the symptoms, perhaps slow its progression, but we can't cure it. To make matters worse, once you have a chronic illness you are more likely to get another one. Chronically ill patients with multiple chronic illnesses represent the rule rather than the exception.

None of these concepts had yet entered my head when I returned from my travels and began my new career as a family physician. It was the 1970s. I was young and had a ponytail, and this image attracted young, healthy people to join the community clinic where I worked as a salaried physician. The clinic was funded by the Ministry of Health and run by a neighbourhood committee consisting of four laypeople from the community. Most of the medical problems I saw were due to acute illness, and the biomedical model that I had been taught worked well. Anything that model didn't understand was explained by stress, and teaching patients the relaxation techniques I had learned from yoga and meditation enhanced my professional reputation within that community. The clinic philosophy involved preventive medicine, educating our patient population, and promoting a healthy lifestyle. We were into wellness before the invention of the word. However, within five years the neighbourhood committee had grown to 15 lay members, and interpersonal conflicts grew accordingly. My colleague and I left what felt like a toxic work environment to start our own practices together. To enhance the services we could provide, we obtained hospital privileges. According to my father, I had finally grown up and the world of conventional medicine was once again a comfortable and stable place for me to work.

My first exposure to environmental medicine was lurking just around the corner. My ensuing curiosity from this experience would lead to criticism, insults, threats, and rejection by many of my colleagues, with subsequent augmentation of my dormant cynicism and frustration. My daughter's birth would add oil to the fire. It would lead to my rejection of the conventional biomedical model and eventual adoption of the biopsychosocial model of health instead.

What is environmental medicine? According to the American Academy of Environmental Medicine, it is the recognition, treatment, and prevention of illnesses induced by exposure to biological and chemical agents encountered in air, food, and water. According to the Canadian Society for Environmental Medicine, it relates to an area of medical practice that concerns medical treatments for individuals who have become ill because of adverse environmental factors such as pollution, and its purpose is to advance the health and well-being of individuals through the improvement of their environment and their relationship to their environment.

More than 80 percent of the patients we see are women aged 30 to 65. These patients have multiple symptoms, involving multiple systems in the body, and usually have no biological markers to aid in the diagnosis. There are no specific abnormalities that show up in blood tests or other diagnostic procedures. The most common organ system involved is the brain, with any or all of five complaints, including fatigue, chronic pain, disturbed sleep, changes in cognition (attention, concentration), and/or mood changes. Upper or lower respiratory complaints and gastrointestinal disturbances (reflux, constipation, diarrhea) are frequent. These patients are more likely to have allergies; food intolerances; sensitivity to some chemical odours (most common is perfume); sensitivity to heat, cold, noise, bright lights, or fluorescent lighting; drug sensitivities; and migraine headaches. They likely have already seen several organ specialists; the good but frustrating news is that no one can find anything wrong. The usual conclusion is that the cause must be stress.

Serendipity

The first time I became aware that environmental factors, other than emotional ones, could induce or influence this pattern of illness occurred shortly after I had left the community clinic to open my own practice. I happened to meet Dr. G., who was working in a clinic run by the most alternative doctor in Ottawa. Everything was treated with vitamins. I was quick to judge him unfairly as weird, and he amplified my perception when he told me that he successfully treated many patients who had arthritis and colitis by diagnosing food allergies. Any physician knows that those problems are not caused by food allergies. On a personal level I am allergic to nuts; exposure puts me in the hospital with a life-threatening reaction. *That's* a food allergy. Confirming my opinion of this doctor was his description of a test he used to aid in the diagnosis: he challenged his patients with different food extracts under the tongue to see if he could provoke a response. It was called a *sublingual challenge test*.

One day Dr. G. confided that he was not happy in the clinic where he worked and was moving out of town. He asked me if he could rent space in my office for a few months before leaving, and I could have his patients after he left. As my partner and I had recently opened the office, we welcomed his contribution to our overhead.

Shortly thereafter, one of my long-time patients, a woman in her early 30s, came for one of her many appointments. She had the symptoms described above, all her tests were normal, she denied emotional stress, and I had run out of specialists to whom I could refer. Her medical chart kept getting thicker. To buy some time, I requested that she change into a gown so that I could do a complete physical and left the room to confer with my partner, because I really didn't know what to do next. Dr. G., a thin, curly-haired man, was perched on the counter with his legs crossed, eating whole-grain wafers covered with some sort of beige spread. He overheard our discussion and exclaimed that she was a textbook case of food allergies; he felt that he could help. I went back into the examination room and told the patient there was a doctor who claimed he could help her. Because of my own skepticism, I advised her that if he didn't help I would reimburse her out of my own pocket, because the tests he wanted to perform were not covered by the provincial health insurance plan. I was also skeptical about the validity and reliability of the sublingual challenge test.

To my surprise, Dr. G. was able to help my patient considerably by placing her on an elimination diet based on the results of the sublingual challenge tests. I was fascinated by what he had accomplished, but shortly thereafter he left town, leaving behind his patients for me to treat. Being unable to treat them according to their needs motivated me to find and attend courses and conferences to learn more. I met the few other doctors in Canada who shared the same interests, and my professional life made a sharp left turn.

By the early 1980s I had a busy family practice. My perception was that it was conventional but that I was open to and supportive of alternative ideas if my patients requested that approach. I taught yoga and meditation techniques to patients who were stressed, or I prescribed tranquilizers and antidepressants when indicated. Conventional or alternative, I bridged the two worlds, and patients who thought they were having reactions to foods continued to seek my services and refer their friends.

I was seeing new patients with chronic complaints more and more frequently. I met with them in small groups in the evenings to test them for possible food sensitivities and then saw them in follow-up to observe their responses to the elimination diets. It seemed that the majority were happy because they felt better, unless they challenged themselves with eliminated foods. But I felt a level of discomfort as I sat on that conventional/alternative fence. I knew that these patients did not have true food allergies according to the definition, yet many of them felt better with the prescribed food-elimination diets.

Allergy or Sensitivity?

The immune system didn't evolve for allergy. Why in a hundred billion years of evolution would we evolve a response for allergy?

— Joel Weinstock

An allergic reaction is an abnormal immune system response to normally harmless environmental substances. The reactions can cause nuisance symptoms, such as itching, or potentially life-threatening responses, such as asthma or anaphylaxis. Frequently these reactions are triggered by harmless everyday substances such as pollen, dust, food, and animal danders. Allergies are not new. In 1873 Charles Blackley, who was a homeopathic physician, demonstrated that the skin of certain individuals with hay fever was sensitive to pollens applied locally to skin that had been abraded. This was the first reported use of the now routine skin-prick test used by all conventional allergists. By the end of the 19th century, investigators had correlated pollen counts with the onset and severity of attacks of hay fever and asthma.

Clemens von Pirquet originally developed the term *allergy* in 1906 from a combination of two Greek words, *allos*, meaning "other," and *ergon*, meaning "reaction." Von Pirquet created the foundation for the modern science of immunology by appreciating that a foreign substance can sensitize: that it can cause an animal to produce a different response to a substance after subsequent exposures. He coined the word *allergy* to describe sensitization, which could be either beneficial, such as developing protection against measles or smallpox, or harmful. When sensitization occurs in reaction to a foreign substance such as pollen or peanuts, it is pathological (abnormal). It is also pathological when we become sensitized to and attack our own tissues, which is known as an autoimmune disease process. A healthy, normal, functioning immune system will recognize all the substances and cells in our own bodies as normal and leave them alone.

Unfortunately, with the passage of time the word *allergy* evolved and is now used to describe only the pathological sensitization to foreign substances. It has become restricted to a limited group of conditions such as hay fever, hives, allergic asthma, allergy to stinging insects, and food anaphylaxis. These disorders almost always involve one immunological response, caused by an antibody called immunoglobulin E, or IgE, which the modern-day skin-prick test used by allergists is very accurate in detecting.

The fact that the term *allergy* is overly restrictive is demonstrated by the fact that clinical allergists treat only selected examples of hypersensitivity states rather than the wide spectrum of immunological disorders. Illogically (or territorially), other hypersensitivity diseases such as celiac disease and contact dermatitis are frequently managed by the relevant organ-based specialists, in these examples, the gastroenterologist and dermatologist. It is the same for the spectrum of autoimmune diseases, including rheumatoid arthritis and lupus (rheumatologists), ulcerative colitis and Crohn's disease (gastroenterologists), multiple sclerosis (neurologists), scleroderma (dermatologists), and glomerulonephritis (nephrologists), just to name a few. Even though all these diseases conform to von Pirquet's original definition of *allergy*, the modern-day allergist does not treat them.

This narrow approach to hypersensitivity by conventional allergists was detrimental to the practice of good medicine. At the beginning, environmental doctors used the term *allergy*, which already existed, though restricted in its definition. This problem could have been overcome by respectful communication, but as will become more apparent, the traditional allergists refused to engage in any respectful dialogue, and so they became the most outspoken and rigid opponents of acceptance of the concepts of environmental medicine. What environmental doctors observed and described was discounted, the doctors were discredited, and the patients were misdiagnosed with psychiatric illnesses, with subsequent prescribing of inappropriate therapies. The allergists were locked in their own box.

CHAPTER 2

FOCUS ON ENVIRONMENTAL MEDICINE

Curiouser and curiouser.

— Lewis Carroll, *Alice's Adventures in Wonderland*

By the mid-1980s my family practice was thriving and I was seeing an increasing number of people for assessment of possible food sensitivities. But another group of symptoms was emerging: some of the patients were claiming to be symptomatic because of exposures to environmental contaminants, especially scented products. They also claimed to have developed a very sensitive sense of smell: they could detect chemical odours when others could not. On one occasion, a patient exclaimed that someone in my office was smoking a cigar, and when she was advised that no one smoked, she refused to accept that fact because she was sure she could smell it. To appease her, I went out into the hallway outside my office and even checked the neighbouring offices down the hall. No one was smoking anything. Nevertheless, she insisted that there was an odour of cigar smoke no one else could detect and that it was provoking her symptoms. To finally prove her wrong, I checked in the office below mine and, to my surprise, the occupant was smoking a cigar. I wondered how anyone could be that sensitive.

The symptoms that these patients claimed were being provoked by chemical exposures were usually subjective, such as:

- ☐ headache
- ☐ mental fatigue
- ☐ irritability
- ☐ nausea
- ☐ shortness of breath
- ☐ cough.

There were no objective physical findings or abnormal tests. Many of the symptoms overlapped with mental disorders such as anxiety. But as I got to know these patients, it was apparent that most of them functioned well unless a chemical exposure was identified; spouses and other family members often supported that observation. Some of them did not function well and were usually symptomatic, even though they attempted to avoid chemical triggers. Why were these patients claiming to react to chemicals at doses they had previously tolerated and that almost everyone else could tolerate? It didn't make sense. For 500 years the mantra of toxicology has been "the dose makes the poison." Were these patients mentally ill?

During my psychiatry rotation in my third year of medical school, they assigned each student a patient from whom to obtain a psychiatric history for discussion. My patient was a delightful 70-year-old man who had been admitted to the hospital's psychiatric unit the previous evening. I asked all the usual questions about mood and psychosocial stresses, but he seemed to be quite normal. He was friendly and behaved appropriately, and I didn't understand why he was there until I eventually asked him. It was 1969. The Front de libération du Québec (FLQ), a terrorist group, had recently bombed the Montreal Stock Exchange. My patient had been persistently calling the Royal Canadian Mounted Police (RCMP) to warn Prime Minister Trudeau that the FLQ was inserting mind-controlling devices into his and other people's brains in order to enhance their revolution. After receiving too many calls, the RCMP brought him to the hospital, where he was admitted with an obvious delusional disorder.

After I presented my case and we had discussed therapy options, I asked what would happen if we gave him a general anesthetic, made a small scalp laceration, put in a few stitches, and then, after he woke up, told him that the device had been removed. The answer was obvious. The device was not the issue. He had a delusional disorder and would most likely be returned to the hospital after a very short time, believing that the device had been reinserted. To pretend to support the delusion would be detrimental, and his new scar would only act as proof.

With this medical school experience in mind, I wondered if I was doing a disservice to patients who claimed to be sensitive to chemicals by being supportive of their perception that chemical pollutants were making them ill and acknowledging their claims of a biological rather than psychological explanation for their illness. And was I also contributing to the illness of those patients with purported food sensitivities? I began to ask all the food-sensitivity patients if they had reactions to chemical odours as well, and many of them responded affirmatively, although they usually found those reactions only mildly bothersome. There seemed to be three types of chemically sensitive patients:

- [ ] those who were mildly sensitive, whose reaction to chemical odours was merely a nuisance
- [ ] those who were significantly sensitive, but avoidance allowed them to otherwise feel and function well. The more sensitive individuals described a rapid onset of more severe symptoms and a more prolonged duration for recovery
- [ ] those who described themselves as very sensitive and who were also chronically unwell, with significant disability. They were more likely to be physically and mentally fatigued and/or have chronic muscular and joint pain.

To learn more, I began to attend annual seminars conducted by the American Society of Clinical Ecology (ASCE). The first one I attended was in 1982 in Banff, where I met several Canadian physicians. Most of the people I encountered were enthusiastic and inquisitive medical practitioners who were either environmentally sensitive themselves or had a close family member with these medical problems. This observation added to my discomfort about sitting on the proverbial fence that divided conventional from alternative medicine. However, what they had to say intrigued me. I attended these meetings annually and found that colleagues from all over North America, England, and Australia were observing the same symptoms of illness that I was. These symptoms were:

- ☐ physical and mental fatigue
- ☐ chronic pain
- ☐ respiratory complaints
- ☐ gastrointestinal complaints
- ☐ rashes
- ☐ allergies
- ☐ food and chemical sensitivities.

These patients had multiple symptoms from multiple body systems, with nothing to be found in the physical exam or laboratory data. I listened to the speakers, many of whom spoke with passion about their observations, and once even sat beside the famous Dr. Linus Pauling. It was at one of these meetings that I first listened to lectures by Dr. Theron Randolph, considered to be the father of environmental medicine.

Mainstream Resistance

Accredited study hours are required to maintain a medical licence. It is important to note that the Accreditation Council for Continuing Medical Education has accredited the seminars conducted by the ASCE, now called the American Academy of Environmental Medicine (AAEM). I point this out because at that time I was also learning that conventional medicine was increasingly and vocally rejecting the AAEM position that people could be sensitive to foods, except via the classical allergic pathway. Even more vehement was the denial that chemical pollutants could be toxic unless there was abnormally high exposure.

As the profile of my medical practice became more apparent to others, I began to note personal rejection by some of my medical colleagues, in particular some of those with whom I shared on-call hospital coverage in evenings and on weekends. I even received a letter suggesting that I reconsider how I was treating these patients, obviously from a concerned colleague, yet sent anonymously.

At the same time I began to witness another emerging clinical phenomenon. In this group of patients, the same symptoms occurred as in those with claims of chemical odour intolerance, but only at the workplace, and perhaps only in a particular room. There were no detectable odours and most of their colleagues had no complaints. The symptoms dissipated when they left that environment and resurged when they returned. Once again there were no physical findings on examination, but if there were enough complaints by co-workers, management would perform indoor air quality assessments. These usually failed to find any significant abnormalities.

In 1984 the World Health Organization (WHO) described this phenomenon — known as sick building syndrome (SBS) — as symptoms that occurred in certain buildings with increased frequency. Note the similarity of the symptoms to those of people complaining of chemical odour sensitivities, multiple symptoms involving the brain, respiratory, and gastrointestinal systems. Symptoms of SBS include:

- ☐ irritation of the eyes, nose, and throat
- ☐ dry, red mucous membranes and skin
- ☐ headache/dizziness
- ☐ upper respiratory infections
- ☐ lower airway symptoms
- ☐ general fatigue
- ☐ nausea.

Despite the WHO's acknowledgement of this phenomenon, reports and opinions began to appear in various medical journals about all these entities. While the opinions were certainly strong, they were also divergent. There were those who described food and chemical sensitivities and sick building syndrome as a physical illness and those who insisted that the illnesses did not exist, that the patients were misattributing symptoms that could be explained only by psychological disorders.

The debate started slowly and gained momentum. Those who felt strongly that the illness was physical were mostly patients, with a few doctors acting as advocates. That the illnesses were psychological dominated mainstream medicine. In 1981 the American Academy of Allergy published a position paper on the techniques advocated and taught by the American Society of Clinical Ecology to diagnose and treat these patients. They stated that sublingual challenge was not reliable as a diagnostic technique, and that no controlled clinical studies demonstrated a therapeutic effect from placing antigens under the tongue.

Resistance to the concepts of what is now called environmental medicine was increasing. This same group of physicians, now called the American Academy of Allergy and Immunology, published a second position statement in 1986.[1] One of the papers cited to support their position was titled "'Allergic to Everything': A Medical Subculture."[2] The author had assessed just eight patients who had filed workers' compensation claims for injury ostensibly caused by an allergic response to substances in the workplace yet who showed no physical evidence of injury. He found the following: withdrawal from work, a lifestyle engineered to avoid exposure to putative noxious substances, and identity as a disabled person. He also observed that they claimed to feel better with austere avoidance of pollutants, such as living in the mountains. The strict environmental

1 "Position Statements: Clinical Ecology. Approved by the Executive Committee of the American Academy of Allergy and Immunology," Journal of Allergy and Clinical Immunology 78, no. 2 (1986): 269–71.
2 C.M. Brodsky, "Allergic to Everything: A Medical Subculture," Psychosomatics 24 (1983): 731–42.

control made them feel and function better, even though they had been diagnosed with psychiatric illness in the past.

Contrast that observation with what I learned in my third year of medical school, when I contemplated pretending to remove the non-existent device from the head of my delusional patient. If sensitivity to environmental factors other than allergy is a psychiatric illness, why did the patients claim to have a better quality of life away from pollutants? The author observed that these patients had found support groups — doctors to diagnose and advise them and lawyers who agreed to help them obtain workers' compensation through litigation. He negatively referred to all this as a "medical subculture." He opined that the patients' perception of an improvement in their quality of life by avoiding chemical triggers was false; it was simply due to this new ideology and the failure of psychiatry to provide explanations. Unfortunately, he concluded that "this subculture seems to appeal to patients with a history of chronic psychiatric symptoms."

It was obvious that the medical community was becoming increasingly polarized regarding the possibility of sensitization to environmental pollutants and foods, and the negative opinion seemed to dominate, especially in the world of allergists. Convinced that they had not reviewed the medical literature fairly or adequately, I continued to practise the same way, until it became evident that my family practice was being overwhelmed.

A Change in Direction

While I may have fallen into environmental medicine by accident, it resulted in my seeing more and more patients with chronic, poorly explained conditions who were being told that their problems were "in their heads." They had a variety of different complaints. Some were helped by an elimination diet; some were helped by reducing exposure to pollutants, especially scented products; some needed therapy for classical allergies; and some needed stress management. What gradually became apparent was that many of them needed more than one of these treatment plans. Most significant was the fact that there were improvements in their health. Many of them became members of my family practice, and I watched the majority function as useful members of society. Most of them worked, maintained close relationships, and raised families. The only difference was that they remained on guard to reduce exposures to identified culprits, whether foods, scented products, pollens, or dust.

My practice became too big and I considered switching to environmental medicine full-time. But what if I was making a mistake? I enjoyed both practices. Would I miss family medicine? I found a recently graduated family medicine physician who was willing to rent my practice, with the idea that each of us would decide after one year whether he would buy it or return it to me.

I had a passion for environmental medicine. It fascinated me to repeatedly witness something they did not teach in medical school and was not within the paradigm of our understanding of disease, yet by listening to patients I could make many feel better. Or could I?

It was now 1985. As the year of renting my practice was coming to an end, it was time to commit to environmental medicine full-time or to return to family medicine. No doubt I had become fascinated with what I thought I was witnessing, but what if I was actually wrong? Was I really helping my patients or was I naive and biased? What if resentment for the disrespectful behaviours of my colleagues was leading me down this path? Unsure and afraid to commit to a possible mistake, I spent a night alone in my office. Perhaps I had been remembering only those who attributed their improvement to my treatments and expressed appreciation. I decided to review 200 consecutive charts to determine as objectively as possible if I was really helping my patients.

Because the presentation of their illnesses varied from one individual to the next, I drew up a list of all the common symptoms and compiled it according to systems, to make it easier to check off. For example, under the heading "gastrointestinal," I listed heartburn, constipation, diarrhea, flatulence, and abdominal bloating. As the sun rose early the next morning, I had tabulated two results. The first confirmed what I had hoped for when I started the previous evening. Seventy percent of the patients reported reduction in frequency and/or severity of at least some symptoms, if not all. I acknowledge that the major criticism of my "study" is that it was poorly designed, with no placebo or control group. This was not a funded study to be published, and my personal bias was not removed, but it was the best way that I could question my instincts. I made my decision — I wanted to sell my family practice.

More important, as I immersed myself in this project, a pattern began to emerge. Most of these patients had symptoms that involved more than one system. Most frequent in the list were complaints of fatigue, decreased concentration, pain, and mood changes. They were not always the main complaint but were present in the history if I asked. If those patients truly had a psychiatric illness, then the elimination of identified foods or avoidance of chemical exposures would not have been helpful in the long run. Just like my delusional patient in medical school, the patients would not have improved, and I would have been contributing to their illnesses.

My young colleague agreed to buy the practice. Excited about my findings, I asked him what he thought about environmental medicine, given that I had diagnosed and treated many of his patients who were environmentally sensitive. To my surprise he stated that he didn't believe in it. When I asked him how he could explain their improvement, he responded, "I don't know what you do behind that door, but I don't believe that it's the prescribed treatments." My attempt to enlighten him with some of the published papers was rebuffed with the statement that he didn't want to talk about it because he hadn't read them. Since that time I have heard from many patients that their doctors do not "believe" in environmental medicine. In science, belief should be based only on good-quality available evidence. At that time, even though medical journals didn't publish many papers on this subject, the medical establishment managed to simply ignore the few available.

CHAPTER 3

EVERYONE'S GOT AN OPINION

Opinion is that exercise of the human will which helps us to make a decision without information.

— John Erskine

On Saturday afternoons I frequently took my family to a neighbourhood toy store owned and run by an enterprising businesswoman. Her husband worked at the cash on weekends and we used to chat. One day he asked me about my medical practice and I described it, including my frustration regarding the issue about whether the illness pattern I was witnessing was psychological or immunological. He asked me what I knew about psychoneuroimmunology, something that I had never heard of and that never appeared in family medicine journals. I now know that psychoneuroimmunology is the study of the communication between the brain and the immune system.

This cashier working for his wife in a toy store on weekends was actually a researcher at the Institute of Neurosciences at Carleton University. He introduced me to the animal experimental literature regarding the multidirectional communication between the immune, autonomic, and central nervous systems. I learned that an antibody response in the body triggers a stress response in the brain, which activates nerve cells to release chemical neurotransmitters. Already four studies had been published that demonstrated this in animals. For the first time I knew the answer to the question of whether the illness pattern we were seeing was physical or mental. The answer was yes.

We take for granted that mental health and emotions affect physical health. For example, it was already well known that emotions could affect immune function and increase the likelihood of getting a cold or aggravating allergies. But the fact that the reverse is also true — that the immune system can affect brain function and that there is a complete circuit between the two systems — was indeed a new concept. Antibodies are molecules that are released in response to a foreign substance. We use them normally to fight infections or, abnormally, in allergic reactions. The animal studies demonstrated that the release of antibodies by the immune system in response to a perceived foreign substance (e.g., a tree pollen) causes a reaction in the brain. This occurs in the same area of the brain, and with the same chemical messengers being released, as when we respond to stress.

Shortly after this encounter, a local allergist asked me to spend an hour with a few medical students to tell them about environmental medicine. He attended as well but did not participate in the discussion. Afterwards I asked him to comment on the recent findings that an immune response could trigger a stress response in the brain. He replied that it was impossible, since the cells of the immune system could not cross the blood–brain barrier. Time, however, has demonstrated that his denial of that possibility was based on faulty reasoning. The cells don't have to cross the blood–brain barrier; they send messages to the brain via the release of chemical messengers.

Informed Opinions

A few years ago I met a young man who was just completing his bachelor of science, majoring in physiology at McGill University, and was applying to medical school. When he was coming down with a cold, his mother recommended that he take vitamin C, an idea he rejected because his

professor claimed there was no evidence that it was effective. I comment-
ed that Linus Pauling, who had been awarded two Nobel Prizes, thought
that it was. The response by this very bright student was that neither of
Pauling's prizes was in medicine.

I went to the medical literature and found the abstracts of two very
recently published studies on the effects of vitamin C on the common
cold. One was favourable and the other was not supportive of positive
effects. I asked him to compare them. The purpose of this exercise was
to demonstrate that these papers, published in peer-reviewed journals,
were still arguing whether vitamin C is beneficial for colds. The argument
had been going on for more than 40 years; opinions simply depended on
how the data was interpreted. I also pointed out to him that, while he was
correct in stating that Pauling's two Nobel Prizes were not in medicine,
the young man's professor at McGill didn't have any.

In the medical literature of the 1960s and 1970s there were many
articles proclaiming the dangers of a vegetarian diet. The *Lancet* is one
of the world's best-known, oldest, and most prestigious peer-reviewed
medical journals. "Peer-reviewed" means that an article has been evaluated and critiqued by researchers and experts in the same field before it
is published. Peer review should ensure that an article maintains a high
standard of quality, accuracy, and academic integrity. However, the *Lancet*
published several very biased papers regarding vegetarian diets. One paper was titled "Death after Vegan Diet."[3] Another, titled "Vegetarianism
and Drug Users," included this prejudicial description:

> . . . hard-core American vegetarians, whose eating habits, as
> well as other aspects of their life-style (e.g., in some cases
> communal or rather casual living arrangements, lack of study,
> work or steady income, and unusual patterns of dress, which
> contrast sharply with that of their parents or peers) distinguish
> them. The diets are bizarre; in addition to simply eliminating
> animal products, most "processed" foods (which they define to

---

3 D. Haler, "Death after Vegan Diet," *Lancet* 292, no. 7560 (1968): 170.

include most canned or frozen foods) are eliminated and extensive use is made of so-called "natural" foods or health foods.[4]

The *Lancet* was and still is one of the most respected medical journals
worldwide, but these papers call attention to the biased frame of reference and transparent lack of objectivity in mainstream medicine at the
time. It was not inappropriate to ask questions regarding potential nutritional deficiencies — such as protein, iron, and vitamin B_{12} — in diets
that eliminate animal products, but well-informed vegetarians compensate accordingly.

Most doctors define mainstream or conventional medicine as what
is taught in medical schools or teaching hospitals. What prestigious journals such as the *Lancet* accept for publication helps define conventional
medicine. Conventional medicine is evidence-based and supported by
good science, while alternative medicine's techniques and treatments are
perceived to be less credible because they have not met the same standards of research, and perhaps never will. Meanwhile, despite the biased
descriptions in the *Lancet*, we now know that vegetarians have lower cholesterol levels and lower rates of high blood pressure and type 2 diabetes than non-vegetarians. Furthermore, vegetarians are less likely to be
overweight and have lower overall cancer rates and mortality rates from
heart disease. History teaches us repeatedly that today's medical gospel
can become tomorrow's old wives' tale.

This *Lancet* discussion shows that, like everyone else, doctors have
opinions that depend on who they are and their own personal biases.
Personal belief systems can also interfere with the interpretation of scientific data. Many medical groups publish position papers. With the potential for bias in mind, we must understand exactly what position papers
are, especially because pure scientific assessments attempt to remove bias.

A position paper is an opinionated report that explains, justifies, or
recommends some particular policy. The literature cited is used to support the authors' position. This is not the same as a systematic literature

---

4 J.T. Dwyer, "Vegetarianism and Drug Users," *Lancet* 298, no. 7739 (1971): 1429–30.

review. A systematic literature review transparently summarizes, classifies, compares, and critically analyzes published research studies, reviews of literature, and theoretical articles. Do not confuse a literature review with a position paper that cites the scientific literature in order to support one view.

Medicine as an Art

Since no two patients are exactly the same, the practice of medicine must also be an art. The art is in being able to make the appropriate diagnosis and choose the correct therapy for each individual from the list of available treatments. There is not always one right answer, and a one-size-fits-all treatment model is not appropriate. Doctors make decisions based on their own clinical experience and their insights, both intuitive and clinical. What works for one patient may not work for the next. There is always a balance between the science of medicine, which attempts to provide consistent evidence-based, almost cookie-cutter, diagnostic and therapeutic techniques, and the personal contribution of the physician, which is the art.

Each physician also brings his own personal flaws to the hospital or clinical exam room. In 2007 the *Journal of General Internal Medicine* reported a study that was designed to examine implicit (unconscious) bias. They studied 220 young emergency medicine residents, in four academic medical centres in Boston and Atlanta, who reported no explicit (conscious) preference for white versus black patients. They used the computer-based Implicit Association Test, which is widely used to measure bias that may not be consciously recognized. This study demonstrated evidence of unconscious racial bias among physicians. The results showed that the physicians' unconscious biases contributed to racial or ethnic disparities in their use of medical procedures for myocardial infarction (heart attack).

Just like those *Lancet* articles on vegetarianism from the sixties, these findings suggest that physicians, just like everybody else, may harbour unconscious preferences and stereotypes that could influence clinical decisions. The good news is that after the study was completed, most of the resident physicians were open to the idea that unconscious biases could affect their clinical decisions, and that learning more about those biases could improve their care of patients. The study has yet to be repeated to confirm the findings, but it emphasizes the point that the personal input of the physician, conscious or not, can potentially influence diagnosis and treatment.

It is not my intention to denigrate my colleagues or my profession, of which I am very proud, but doctors are no different from laypeople in being influenced by their personal and cultural characteristics during decision-making. We require critical self-reflection, ego control, and the ability to change in order not to fail at the art of healing. Science is supposed to be self-correcting and to modify according to emerging data, but those who are doctrinaire are very slow to change. While this is not unique to medicine, the fact remains that some of the early observations being made by environmental physicians could not be explained by existing paradigms. If people were really being made sick by their environment, those paradigms were wrong and the opponents were being doctrinaire.

More Resistance

In 1981 the California Medical Association (CMA) adopted the position that clinical ecology, now known as environmental medicine, did not constitute a valid medical discipline and that scientific and clinical evidence to support the diagnosis of environmental illness was lacking. In 1984, as a result of requests from clinical ecologists for endorsement, the CMA appointed a task force to conduct a hearing at which the proponents of clinical ecology could present their views, provide pertinent literature for review, and formulate recommendations to the CMA. The task force addressed three main questions:

☐ Are there certain symptoms or signs that might allow physicians to identify specific diseases or syndromes induced by low-level environmental exposure as defined by clinical ecologists?

☐ Do reliable tests exist that provide objective evidence of such diagnoses?

☐ Are there proven therapies that are beneficial for patients who have been identified as having symptoms related to environmental exposure?

The task force's conclusions were as follows:

☐ There is no convincing evidence that supports the hypotheses on which clinical ecology is based

☐ Clinical ecologists have not identified specific, recognizable diseases caused by exposure to low-level environmental stressors

☐ Methods to diagnose and treat such unidentified conditions have not been shown to be effective.

This took place in the 1980s, and at that time not a lot of evidence was available. What is disconcerting is that the panel roundly criticized the papers presented to the CMA by the proponents, while no faults or criticisms were identified for the two papers contrary to the clinical ecology viewpoint. One study, published in the *Archives of Internal Medicine*, described 50 patients who had been diagnosed with multiple chemical sensitivities (MCS) and had been unsuccessfully treated by clinical ecologists. The author was an allergist who found there were no abnormalities either on physical examination or in laboratory tests — which we know is typical.

The study claimed to examine treatment failures. However, half of the patients did not even have the correct pattern of illness. Most of them had constant symptoms, even when they were avoiding chemicals. This is inconsistent with the concept that the symptoms of multiple chemical sensitivities are provoked by exposure to chemicals. Clearly the author did not understand the nature of the disorder. He assessed poorly chosen subjects who had been unsuccessfully treated and then concluded that people could not become ill from exposure to chemicals.

The panel accepted this paper without any criticism, sitting in judgment of something that they did not or refused to understand. There was bias in favour of the science presented to them by the opponents of clinical ecology. They narrowly focused on the diagnostic tests and treatments used to try to desensitize the patients. They did not recognize that there was an evolving illness pattern that was unique, and they discredited patients who were truly suffering from environmental sensitivities.

A Crack in the Resistance Wall

After receiving numerous complaints from Canadian patients about their reactions to chemicals in the environment and the lack of support and acknowledgement by the medical profession, in November 1984 the Ministry of Health for the province of Ontario established an ad hoc committee chaired by Judge George Thomson. The committee's mandate was to determine whether environmental hypersensitivity, which was the term the committee preferred, really existed. To assess the knowledge of the disorder available at that time, the committee invited briefs and submissions (it received 1,209), met with professional and patient groups, and consulted with experts in several fields. Some members of the committee visited U.S. environmental control units where clinical ecology treatment was offered in an institutional setting. The committee members also met with most of Ontario's clinical ecologists, including spending an afternoon in my office.

The 314-page report was tabled before the Ontario legislature in December 1985. The committee stated that it was "impressed by the calibre of medicine practised by some of the doctors" who tried to treat the patient as a partner in diagnosis and treatment. The committee noted, however, that scientifically unproven testing and treatment methods had found wide acceptance, and that some practitioners were willing to adopt new techniques that lacked even theoretical explanations.

The clinical ecologists testified that a healthy body is not normally troubled by low levels of chemicals, but under the stress of a triggering event it may become unable to handle the combined effects of different substances. The committee noted that this "total load" concept of additive effects had the attraction of logic but there was no experimental support for its role in environmental hypersensitivity. The committee became convinced that emotional and psychological factors play a role in some patients, but it could not say to what extent this contributed to the overall problem.

It became clear that careful history-taking was a very important tool in the diagnosis of environmental hypersensitivities. The genuine attention given to the patient's story was regarded as such a positive point that the committee recommended recognizing the extra time involved in the Ontario Hospital Insurance Plan (OHIP) fee schedule. But it took more than 30 years before the system in Ontario was restructured to allow billing for the extra time required to assess and treat chronic complex medical conditions like these.

The conclusion the committee reached after all its reading, discussion, and observation was that it had found good reason to believe that some people suffer adverse effects from environmental factors, in ways not accounted for by immunologic or toxicologic knowledge. It was the committee's opinion that the diagnosis of environmental hypersensitivity had validity.

Its report recommended the establishment of an environmental control unit in Ontario that would care for the province's most disabled patients and facilitate the spread of balanced information among both the public and professionals. The unit would also provide the expertise and the controlled environment necessary for reliable research. This eventually led to development of the Environmental Hypersensitivity Research Unit (EHRU) at the University of Toronto in 1994 and the collaborating Environmental Health Clinic, established at Women's College Hospital, a teaching hospital associated with the medical school of the University of Toronto. Although I worked in Ottawa, I began collaborating with them immediately.

PART II

WHAT'S MAKING US SICK

CHAPTER 4

OUTDOOR AIR

In an underdeveloped country, don't drink the water; in a developed country, don't breathe the air.

— Jonathan Raban

People with environmental sensitivities describe themselves as canaries in a coal mine. This refers to the old mining tradition described in the introduction to this book, in which miners used canaries to warn them that toxic gases were accumulating. Environmentally sensitive patients have become more sensitive to lower levels of chemical pollutants than other people. But are they really canaries? Can it be possible that the rest of us are also at risk from incessant but low-level chemical pollutant exposures? If so, where's the evidence?

People are aware that there is a problem with outdoor air pollution without really understanding how it is changing our health. Since the increase in pollution, many chronic illnesses are increasing in incidence. Neurodegenerative disorders such as Parkinson's and Alzheimer's disease are on the rise. So are immune disorders such as allergies, asthma, and autoimmune diseases, including Crohn's disease, lupus, and endometriosis. There are more deaths and hospital admissions on "bad air" days. Accompanying the increase in pollution are newly emerging diseases such as chronic fatigue syndrome (ME/CFS), and people with these conditions are often environmentally sensitive as well.[5]

Patients with environmental sensitivities find that their symptoms are provoked by chemical pollutant exposures at levels they previously tolerated and that are tolerated by the normal population. For these people, the effect of chemical exposures is clear. The premise of this book, supported by several thousand studies in the medical literature, is that there is a link between chronic illness and chemical exposures. The link is our biological inability to handle them, even if we can't feel it. Maybe we should listen to these canaries.

The Chemical Soup

Since the Second World War, approximately 80,000 new synthetic chemicals have been manufactured and released into the environment, with approximately 1,500 new chemicals being introduced every year. The vast majority of these have not been adequately tested for their impacts on human health or their particular impacts on children and the developing fetus. Some chemicals are mass produced and known as "high production volume" chemicals, meaning that annual production and/or importation volumes are above one million pounds. In the United States it is estimated that up to 7.1 trillion pounds of these chemicals are produced or imported annually. Basic toxicity information is available for less than 50 percent of these, and information on developmental toxicity is available for less than 20 percent.

The Organisation for Economic Co-operation and Development (OECD), which has 34 member countries, has maintained a list of

---

5 The term *chronic fatigue syndrome* (CFS) is most often used by doctors in North America. This is because the main symptom is often fatigue and the condition is chronic (persistent). Many people prefer the term *myalgic encephalomyelitis* (ME) because the word *fatigue* does not reflect the severity and difference in character of the fatigue. Some believe that there are two separate conditions, CFS and ME, but the medical literature usually refers to CFS and ME as the same entity. I will use the umbrella term *ME/CFS*.

5,235 high-production-volume chemicals since 2000. The OECD list includes all chemicals that have annual production volumes greater than 1,000 tonnes (2.2 million pounds) in more than one economically developed country. A large number of these chemicals are in our food, water, and air.

Pollutants in the Air

Almost 80 percent of the people in Canada and the United States live in urban communities with varying levels of air pollution. Urban air pollution comes predominantly from burning fossil fuels, which include coal, oil, and gas. Greenhouse gases are not the only pollutants produced by the burning of fossil fuels. Coal-fired plants and other fossil-fuel burners produce other gases, such as nitrogen oxides, sulphur dioxide, and volatile organic compounds (VOCs). These all contribute to production of the chemical soup. Fossil fuel burning and other industrial processes also add heavy metals, such as mercury, and fine particulate matter — small, discrete masses of solid or liquid that remain individually dispersed in the air.

Fossil fuel burning is used to produce energy for transportation, factories, heating buildings and water, and production of electricity. Other polluting gases come from decomposing garbage in landfills and solid-waste disposal sites, and many household products release VOCs. All these chemicals constitute a very diverse group of substances, many of which can be toxic. Some may degrade slowly and persist in the environment for years.

Chemical pollutants tend to degrade at different rates. They exist in solid, liquid, or gas phases and, just like water, can switch from one phase to another depending on the temperature. Some simply break down or degrade quite quickly, some mix with other chemicals to form new ones, and others degrade more slowly. Some pollutants are quite resistant to degradation and break down so slowly that they are labelled "persistent organic pollutants" (POPs). As they disperse into the atmosphere, many chemicals are capable of travelling long distances, depending on how long they stay suspended in the air, floating in the wind. Some pollutants quickly fall to the ground because of gravity, some get pulled from the sky when it rains or snows, and many others are dispersed rapidly and directly on nearby land. If they don't decay quickly, they eventually get into the water table below the surface of the ground. Many end up in major waterways and ultimately the oceans, whose currents then help spread the contaminants around the world.

The longer they persist, the more prone pollutants are to long-range transport. Scientists classify them as flyers, hoppers, and swimmers, depending on how they disperse. Flyers stay in the air for long periods and swimmers are transported via the waterways of the world. Most POPs are multi-hoppers, bouncing around the planet according to the wind and weather. Temperature can also affect the movement of these chemicals. Lower temperatures tend to convert the compounds into larger particles; this increases the likelihood that rain and snow will remove the particles from the atmosphere, transporting them to the surface of the earth. Because many of these chemicals persist for long periods of time in the environment, they can bioaccumulate, meaning that they can be absorbed by and accumulate in living organisms, and as they do so, they are passed from one species to the next, up the food chain.

In chemistry, *organic* does not mean that the chemical substance is free of pesticides and other man-made substances. Chemists begin their classification of chemicals by dividing them into two groups, organic and inorganic. *Organic* means that the chemicals contain carbon as part of their basic molecular structure. Most organic pollutants are soluble in oil, and because fat is oil in a solid form, they tend to accumulate in fats, especially if they resist biodegradation. (This will become an important point when we review how to minimize the dangers of these chemicals to our health.) The higher an organism is in the food chain, the greater the accumulation. We humans sit at the top of the food chain, consuming the animals below us, including their fat.

Does direct exposure to outdoor air pollution have any effects on human health? We have been studying this for years. In the 1960s epidemiologists, or scientists who study the patterns of health and disease, considered these issues. The epidemiology studies produced back then appeared to lack the sensitivity to detect increases in cancers, significant mortality, or morbidity from air pollution exposures. However, the science of epidemiology has continued to evolve, and its ability to finesse and assess patterns of disease has improved considerably. For example, we now know that outdoor air pollution has a considerable impact on mortality and cardiopulmonary disease.

WHO Is Asking

Thresholds are concentrations below which effects are not observed, either in the general population or in selected susceptible populations (e.g., the elderly or children). Toxicologists measure thresholds. According to a World Health Organization (WHO) report published in 2003, there are several unanswered questions regarding thresholds and risk:

- ☐ Does the latest evidence in toxicology even support the concept of thresholds?
- ☐ Is there a threshold for individual chemicals below which no effect on health is expected to occur in all people?
- ☐ In the absence of a threshold, what is required for the development of standards to provide an "acceptable level of risk"?
- ☐ What is an acceptable level of risk?

That same report noted the following issues:

- ☐ Increasingly better and more sensitive epidemiological study designs have identified adverse effects from air pollution at much lower levels of exposure than previously thought.

☐ Thresholds differ, depending on the outcome selected. They depend on:

- the endpoint chosen (e.g., death, diminished pulmonary function, molecular changes);
- the nature of the population being assessed (e.g., from the healthiest to the most ill, healthy male or pregnant female, child versus adult);
- the time at which the response is measured (e.g., immediate response versus delayed, accumulated exposures over time).

☐ For some pollutants, adverse health effects are expected at low levels in susceptible people (e.g., asthmatics), even where present air quality standards are being met.

☐ Epidemiological studies are limited in their ability to detect thresholds.

☐ Toxicological studies are also limited.

Lack of evidence for an adverse health effect from a chemical does not mean that there is no health effect. It might just mean that it hasn't been found yet. According to the WHO, "the absence of evidence is not the same as evidence of absence."

Major Contributors

There are six "criteria" air pollutants for which the U.S. Environmental Protection Agency (EPA) has established National Ambient Air Quality Standards under the *Clean Air Act*. These are defined as commonly found air pollutants that can cause harm to health and the environment and cause property damage. They are:

☐ particulate matter
☐ ozone

- ☐ nitrogen oxides
- ☐ sulphur oxides
- ☐ carbon monoxide
- ☐ lead.

Particulate matter, ozone, and nitrogen oxides are the major contributors to outdoor air pollution. Of the six pollutants, studies have identified two as the most widespread health threats: particulate matter and ground-level ozone. Ozone is formed naturally in the atmosphere, where it serves an important purpose: blocking the sun's ultraviolet rays, which can cause cancer. At ground level it is poisonous. Trying to study which pollutants are unsafe, and at which levels, is difficult because the reality is that air pollution is a complex mixture. The influence of the pollutants could be additive or synergistic — each one makes the other(s) more toxic.

It is now very clear that adverse health effects are associated with pollution in most urban centres. Governments gather accurate statistics for mortality and morbidity as measured by death certificates, visits to emergency departments, and admissions to hospitals, including intensive care units. The studies of air-quality effects on health demonstrate unequivocally that increased air pollution is associated with increased rates of visits to doctors, hospitalization, and premature death.

Exposure to outdoor particulate matter (PM) is responsible for a significant amount of mortality from cardiopulmonary disease, lung cancer, and acute respiratory infection in children living in urban areas worldwide. Air pollution can exacerbate symptoms in persons with lung diseases such as asthma and chronic obstructive pulmonary disease (COPD). What is surprising, however, is that poor air quality does not affect only patients with respiratory conditions.

Exposure to PM correlates with higher blood concentrations of oxidized low-density lipoprotein (LDL), which is the "bad cholesterol" associated with potential cardiovascular disease and with atherosclerosis, in which the walls of arteries are filled with plaques of fat. Cardiovascular disease includes hardening of the arteries, high blood pressure, heart disease, and stroke. According to the American Heart Association, exposure to outdoor air PM over a few hours to a few weeks can trigger fatal heart attacks and strokes, as well as non-fatal events. Longer-term exposure increases the risk for cardiovascular mortality to an even greater extent, and it reduces life expectancy by up to a few years in those who are more heavily exposed. Although results differ among studies, there is also increasing evidence for a relationship between air pollution exposure and elevated blood pressure levels. Regarding stroke, the long-term chance for survival after a stroke is lower among patients who live in areas with higher levels of outdoor air pollution.

We are also seeing more allergies with greater severity, and these changes are associated with air pollution exposure. Children are particularly vulnerable to the effects of outdoor air pollution. Those who live in urban areas have higher rates of allergy compared with those from rural areas. Numerous studies demonstrate the increased likelihood of wheezing, asthma, and allergic rhinitis in kids who have more pollution exposure. Several studies also show adverse effects of outdoor air pollutants on lung development in children of all ages. In one study, children were followed from age 10 to 18; those who lived less than 500 metres from major roadways were compared with those who lived more than 1,500 metres away. Close proximity to traffic resulted in reduced lung-function growth over the eight-year period, and deficits in lung function at age 18.

Numerous other studies emphasize that close proximity to street traffic is associated with more childhood allergies and asthma. Clearly, living closer to major traffic increases pollutant exposure and puts people of all ages at risk. In 2002 the *Lancet* published a study of 5,000 people aged 55 to 69 who lived near a major road; they were followed for eight years. It revealed that they had double the risk for death from cardio-pulmonary causes. Since that *Lancet* study, other studies have compared people living within 300 metres of a major road to those living much farther away. A literature review of 29 studies also revealed increased risk of preterm births, allergies, asthma, respiratory infections, and impaired cardiovascular function.

"Major traffic" is defined as 10,000 cars per day. You can find out the traffic statistics for your municipality. How close are you?

Particulates That Matter

The heat from sunlight aids in producing ozone, so it is usually higher in the summer than in the winter. Smog is produced when we mix ground-level ozone with particulate matter in the air.

Particulate matter is made from a mixture of pollutants and is a by-product of the combustion of fossil fuels. It is measured in units called microns; a micron is equal to 0.001 millimetre or 0.000039 inch. To put the size of a micron into perspective, when the sun shines through the window at just the right angle, you can see some particulate matter floating in the air in your house. The smallest size that one can see with the naked eye is 50 microns — the head of a pin or the thickness of a human hair.

There are three categories of particulate matter, according to size:

- ☐ *Coarse* particulates (2.5–10 microns, or PM_{10}) are usually filtered by the hairs and cilia of our upper respiratory systems
- ☐ *Fine* particulate matter (less than 2.5 microns, or $PM_{2.5}$) gets into the small bronchial tubes or alveoli (the tiny sacs where air exchange takes place)
- ☐ *Ultrafine* particulate matter (less than 0.1 micron) is so small that it can penetrate inside the body, and even inside cells.

Studies in rats demonstrate that ultrafine particulate matter can be transferred directly to the brain from the mucous lining of the nose, via the olfactory (sense of smell) nerve. A study was made of healthy children and young adults in Mexico City who had died suddenly as a result of accident or suicide. Their autopsies found PM in higher amounts in the brain, in particular the root of the olfactory nerve, when compared to controls from two cities with very low pollution levels. Mexico City has high levels of air pollution, and children who live there are more likely to have MRI brain scan abnormalities. Similar lesions have been found in dogs from the same city. When they were sacrificed, ultrafine particulate matter deposits were found in their brains.

Air Quality Index

Where you live makes a difference, both regionally and locally. An example of pollution that travels from region to region is demonstrated in Toronto, Ontario. The prevailing winds usually come from Michigan and Ohio, where there is significant coal burning. These winds assist in transferring that pollution for long distances, contributing to the polluted air found in Toronto.

Aside from moving to the top of a mountain or purchasing your own island in the Pacific, there are ways for you to minimize the risk of outdoor air exposure. A daily air quality reading, called the Air Quality Index, is available on TV weather channels and the internet for most municipalities in North America and Europe. It is limited to PM_{10} and $PM_{2.5}$ particulate matter, ground-level ozone, and nitrogen oxide, and each pollutant is assigned a number from 0 to 500. The Air Quality Index reports only the highest pollutant score for that day. It does not consider multiple exposures and is not very accurate as a measure for health risk.

Air Quality Health Index

We are getting better at measuring and understanding the risks of outdoor pollution exposure and can now provide some advice to minimize the impact, especially for those who we know are at increased risk. In

2011 Canada began a pilot project using a different scale, the Air Quality Health Index (AQHI), which is based on measured risk for adverse health effects. It considers the mixture of pollutants and shows the relative health risk associated with the total air pollution level. The index is designed to help people understand what air quality means to health. Using a scale from 1 to 10+, it shows the relative health risk associated with the total air pollution level. We use this scale to warn people who are at risk to reduce their outdoor activities. The higher the value of the AQHI, the more likely it is that people will experience symptoms associated with poor air quality.

The AQHI website states: "Air pollution makes it even harder for people to breathe and can make existing lung or heart-related symptoms worse. For example, it can trigger heart attacks." Those at risk are identified as:

☐ people who have existing respiratory illnesses such as asthma, COPD (which includes chronic bronchitis and emphysema), or lung cancer;
☐ those with existing cardiovascular conditions such as angina, previous heart attack, congestive heart failure, or heart rhythm problems (arrhythmia or irregular heartbeat);
☐ people with diabetes, because they are more likely to have cardiovascular disease.

The medical literature recognizes the negative effect of outdoor air pollution on these diseases, but what is the mechanism? Does it have anything to do with the message from the canaries? Is the impact only on people who are already ill? And there are other chemicals that we are all exposed to that are also a burden to our bodies. The canaries are warning us of the dangers of those too, while at the same time industry and traditional toxicologists are reassuring us that our levels of exposures are safe. So who is right? Does it make good sense for everyone else to also decrease exposures to these chemical pollutants?

CHAPTER 5

THE BODY BURDEN

What is our minimum daily requirement for Teflon?
— David Wineberg

Here's an idea for an experiment. Let's take 200 different medications, empty all the capsule contents into a container, mix it up, and then swallow a capsule full of this mixture every day to see what happens. Why not? It's just a very low dose of 200 different medications. Better yet, maybe we should try this experiment on our children. Even more interesting would be to have expectant mothers take this concoction every day during pregnancy to see what might happen to their unborn babies.

Thankfully, because of the obvious risk of serious harm, no ethics committee in any research facility would ever approve such an experiment, but given the option, would you volunteer to participate? Unbeknownst to you, a similar experiment has been going on for more than 30 years — but it's not being conducted by the drug industry. The average North American body contains up to 200 different environmental pollutants. We call this the body burden.

Gathering the evidence for this began in the early 1980s, when the U.S. Environmental Protection Agency looked for evidence of human environmental contamination by obtaining fat samples from cadavers and specimens removed in surgery. More than 700 chemical substances were found to be stored in the fat tissue of the general American population. Since then, the U.S. Centers for Disease Control (CDC) have published four studies of chemical body burdens, showing that North Americans carry as many as 212 contaminants in their bodies, and that women have higher levels of many of those chemicals than men do. We all have most of these chemicals stored in our bodies because we keep on ingesting them and/or because we can't break them down.

National Health and Nutrition Examination Surveys

The Environmental Health Laboratory at the CDC published its first report, called the *National Health and Nutrition Examination Survey (NHANES I)*, in 1991. The researchers measured 27 chemicals in humans. After looking for more, their second report, *NHANES II* (1999–2000), contained data for 116 environmental chemicals. One positive note was that it showed improvement in some areas due to decrease or discontinuation of use of some pollutants, such as lead, which had been banned as an additive in gasoline products. Synthetic musks, however, which are commonly used in fragrances — including in cleaning products, detergents, and personal care products — have at least tripled in human breast milk during the past decade.

Exposure data on an additional 32 chemical pollutants were published in *NHANES III* (2005). These additional chemicals include insecticides, herbicides, pesticides, plastics, polychlorinated biphenyls (PCBs), dioxins, furans, and polycyclic aromatic hydrocarbons from the burning of fossil fuels. Seventy-five more chemicals were added to the list in the fourth report, *NHANES IV* (2009). The data reveal that 99 percent of the population have fire retardants in their bodies and 90 percent of the population have plastics. Most people also contain pesticides, heat-resistant non-stick coatings (such as Teflon), stain-resistant chemicals, industrial chemicals, heavy metals, and more. And we don't even know how to test the additive or synergistic effects of these 200-plus different chemicals.

Other Published Reports

In 2010 Health Canada published its own human biomonitoring report. Researchers measured 91 chemicals, including heavy metals, organochlorines, PCBs (banned, but a persistent pollutant), PFCs (stain repellents), phthalates (plastics), bisphenol A (BPA), pesticides, chlorphenols (antiseptics), and tobacco smoke. Cotinine reflects intake of tobacco smoke. What is disturbing about cotinine is that it is still being found in Canadian non-smokers, although the levels have decreased since the bans on smoking in public places.

Some independent groups have obtained private funding and published their own data. Environmental Defence Canada published its *Toxic Nation* report in 2005. Researchers tested for 88 chemicals in 11 volunteers and detected 60 different pollutants. The average volunteer contained 44 of the chemicals tested. But most disconcerting is the work of the Environmental Working Group, an American advocacy group. In 2005 and 2009, it did two small studies of 10 American, Canadian, and Dutch newborn babies, in which researchers measured the chemicals found in cord blood, taken from the blood vessels of the cut umbilical cord immediately after the babies were born. In both studies they found well over 200 chemicals in the newborn babies. This group has performed 11 studies to date and has found 414 industrial chemicals, pollutants, and pesticides in 186 people, from newborns to grandparents. More than 400 publications are available in the U.S. National Library of Medicine that confirm the presence of pollutants in unborn children.

What has been the chemical industry's response to these studies? When the *NHANES IV* report on the human body burden of chemical pollutants was released in 2009, the American Chemistry Council, not surprisingly, immediately responded with the following spin:

> The American Chemistry Council (ACC) and its member companies reiterate their support for the U.S. Centers for Disease Control and Prevention's (CDC) scientific efforts to

understand human exposure to natural and man-made substances through biomonitoring. Like the previous three studies, the 4th CDC report reaffirms that levels of man-made and natural compounds detected in Americans remain low.

Processing the Information

What's wrong with this human experiment?

☐ It is unethical because there is risk of damage that could be permanent.

☐ There is no informed consent. Who gave permission to fill us up with chemicals without our knowledge? Few people are aware and no one was ever given a choice.

☐ There is no control group — no one who is not heavily contaminated — so we don't have a population to compare ourselves with in order to look for possible health impacts. Everyone has chemicals in them. The only way that we can study the impact of the 200 body-burden chemicals on health is to try to find people with higher exposure and compare them to people who have less exposure. This is like doing a study comparing people who smoke a pack of cigarettes per day to people who smoke half a pack; if both groups get cancer, you can't see a difference. The smokers need to be compared to non-smokers. Without a good control group of unexposed subjects for comparison, finding adverse health effects is more difficult.

☐ We do not have the ability to study the potential impact of several hundred different chemical exposures that occur at the same time but vary from one individual to another.

☐ The funding for this experiment comes from the health care system and we, the consumers, propagate the experiment with our lifestyle. What have we learned from it so far?

☐ Biomonitoring can estimate how much of a chemical is present in a person, but we cannot tell what health effects, if any, may result from single or multiple exposures.

☐ The absence of a chemical does not necessarily guarantee that the person has not been exposed. It may only mean that it was not present inside the body at the time the test was taken.

☐ Biomonitoring cannot determine the source of the exposure or its route of entry into the body.

☐ Most significant is that we do not know whether some or all of these chemicals have an additive or multiplying effect.

The chemical industry remains confident that no harm is being done, because the levels of their production by-products found in humans remain low.

What is obvious from the bioaccumulation information gathered is that we are regularly exposed to a variety of hazardous chemicals and constantly carry varying levels of many of them in our bodies. They can be found throughout the body, including in blood serum, semen, fat, bone, the follicular fluid in which eggs reside in the ovaries, and breast milk, and females tend to have higher levels than males. Unknowingly, women marinate their eggs and baste and incubate their unborn children in 200 chemical pollutants, after which they feed them to their babies. It doesn't matter whether it's breast milk or cow's milk — both are polluted. More than 90 percent of our pollutant exposures come from sources that are close to us and within our control, although we do not realize it, and most are from sources that are not regulated — they are not controlled by law.

Are you reassured by the ACC's insistence that we need not worry about our children's health, because the levels of chemical exposures remain low? Many chronic illnesses have increased in incidence since the increase in pollution, including neurodegenerative disorders, immune, cardiovascular, and respiratory diseases, and developmental disorders in children. This and the new, emerging illnesses such as FM, ME/CFS, and

MCS raise questions as to whether and how such divergent conditions are related to pollution:

- [ ] Is there a cause-and-effect relationship?
- [ ] If there is, what is the mechanism?
- [ ] If the exposures of individual chemical pollutants are too low to be toxic, as claimed by the chemical industry and opponents of the existence of SBS and MCS, why are the incidences increasing?
- [ ] Why are so many divergent disease patterns occurring, given that we all seem to experience the same burden of pollution exposure?
- [ ] Why can't we just degrade and/or excrete the body burden of pollutants?
- [ ] None of the individual chemical levels are considered high enough to be toxic, but what about the "soup"? Is it not possible that it may cause numerous interactions and unpredicted changes in how we feel and function?

The traditional "the dose makes the poison" mantra of toxicologists supports the American Chemistry Council's position that our exposure levels are safe. Epidemiologists have observed negative changes in patterns of many chronic illnesses that they associate with increases in pollution exposure. This raises the question as to whether there is a cause-and-effect relationship between these exposures and adverse health effects. One of the requirements to determine the significance of an association is whether the association observed makes scientific sense. The traditional toxicology mantra tells us that it does not. If that 500-year-old paradigm is wrong, where's the evidence?

Most chronic illnesses begin insidiously and gradually. How can it happen that a person drops dead five minutes after leaving the doctor's office, confident that he is healthy? Subtle, clinically immeasurable changes, which may occur over long periods, slowly lead to changes in homeostasis, or balance. The result can be either an abrupt change (such as sudden death) or gradual deterioration, which is chronic illness. Eventually organ malfunction develops and the changes are then measurable, which helps direct the physician to diagnose a recognizable, clinically apparent disease. *You had a heart attack. Your mother has developed Parkinson's disease. Your child now has asthma. You have cancer.* The universal response is always the same: *How did this happen? What can I do about it now? Is it too late? What is my prognosis?* Why weren't the changes leading up to the illness apparent in tests performed in the doctor's office or clinical laboratory? If all our tests suggest that the organ involved is okay until the disease shows up, where should we look for evidence that something is occurring that will eventually change the balance?

Methods and suggestions to reduce the body burden are described in later chapters. But before delving into the solutions, it is important to understand how the environment is actually affecting our health. In the previous chapter, I discussed the impact of bad air days on people's health. One might think that staying indoors would reduce our risk of exposure. But does it?

CHAPTER 6

INDOOR AIR

There is nothing like staying at home for real comfort.

— Jane Austen

In the 1970s, there was an oil embargo and the price of oil skyrocketed. Higher energy prices led to the construction of tighter buildings, which seemed like a good idea because it also meant less contamination from outdoor air pollution. However, the reduced ventilation also meant that less indoor air was leaving the indoor environment.

The world's economic response to the energy crisis was inflation. Everything became more expensive, which led to the widespread use of cheaper manufactured building materials. Linoleum, vinyl, and synthetic carpets replaced hardwood floors, and composites replaced natural wood. Composite wood products, such as particleboard and medium-density fibreboard (MDF), are made from wood fibre and glues. They are widely used in the manufacturing of furniture, kitchen cabinets, doors, mouldings, window casings, baseboards, and laminate flooring. These new indoor materials slowly release small amounts of chemical vapours ("off-gassing"), notably VOCs, into the indoor environment. So at the same time that we reduced the ventilation of our buildings, we increased their indoor contamination, making indoor air more polluted than outdoor air.

By the late 1970s there was already an awareness of indoor air pollution. The EPA found that the levels of common organic pollutants were two to five times higher inside homes than outside, regardless of whether the homes were located in rural or highly industrial areas. Many other studies have supported the findings that chemical pollutant exposure is much higher indoors. Given that Americans, Canadians, and Europeans spend 90 percent of their time indoors, questions are continuously being raised regarding the significance of these exposures and their potential impact on human health.

The amount of time we spend in a particular location and the activities that occur there are important factors to consider when studying the effects of indoor air exposures. There are also other reasons why individual exposures differ. A study of patterns of exposure in seven European regions, which differed by culture rather than by weather, found that the following factors influenced the amount of time individuals spend in different indoor environments:

- age
- gender
- different weather variables
- day type (weekend, weekday, vacation, etc.)
- lifestyle and life stage considerations, which in turn are influenced by
  - type of work
  - employment status
  - season
- living alone, having children at home (raising children leads to adapting schedules and to more time being spent at home and less at work and in other indoor places).

Indoor Air Quality

The air quality in spaces designed for occupancy should be defined by its effect on humans. Most important, the air we breathe indoors should not have a negative effect on our health and it should be perceived as acceptable or even better — fresh and pleasant. We want indoor air to have a positive impact on our work performance and our productivity, and we do not want the air quality in the classroom to interfere with our children's academic performance. How do we meet these requirements?

Since we know that it is the chemicals emitted by people, materials, and processes that decrease the indoor air quality (IAQ), why can't we just make sure that the concentration of each chemical in the air is below a certain guideline value? The answer is that there are typically hundreds of chemicals in the indoor air, each in very small concentrations, and we have limited information on their impact on health and comfort. Guideline values are available for only a few dozen chemicals, and they apply only when the exposure occurs to each alone.

We know the odour or irritation levels for a large number of chemicals, so maybe we should use them instead of waiting for information on health effects. Unfortunately, the thresholds for some chemicals vary considerably from person to person. Thresholds tell us the concentration at which 50 percent of people can perceive that specific chemical when it occurs alone. However, the most sensitive people can perceive the same chemical at a concentration that is several orders of magnitude lower, and they may notice a cocktail of hundreds of chemicals at even lower concentrations. Furthermore, some chemicals, even though above an odour threshold, may be perceived as pleasant, while others may seem very unpleasant. A further obstacle is that many chemicals are difficult to measure in the very small concentrations at which they may still have a negative impact on people.

Pollution at Home

When you buy a house, your realtor and lawyer will tell you to get a building inspection done before the deal is closed. But you should be aware that, according to their standards of practice, a qualified building inspector is not required or expected to determine the quality of the air or to identify air contaminants. To do this kind of assessment requires a building engineer, who is trained and equipped to do the required testing and evaluate the significance of the results according to established guidelines and standards. These standards are produced by the American Society of Heating, Refrigerating and Air-Conditioning Engineers (ASHRAE). ASHRAE is now an international organization that provides standards for the design and maintenance of indoor environments.

According to ASHRAE, acceptable indoor air quality is defined as "air in which there are no known contaminants at harmful concentrations as determined by cognizant authorities and with which a substantial majority (80 percent or more) of the people exposed do not express dissatisfaction." So if 19 percent of the inhabitants of a building complain about the IAQ, it is still acceptable. The tighter the building structure is, the more responsibility the ventilation has for "breathing for us"; it must bring in the oxygen and exhaust the carbon dioxide. ASHRAE also states that "comfort criteria, with respect to human bioeffluents (odour), are likely to be satisfied if the ventilation results in indoor carbon dioxide concentrations less than 700 parts per million above the outdoor air concentration." In other words, the criterion for human comfort is that you can't smell your family or colleagues.

If the ventilation is inadequate, the carbon dioxide level indoors will increase. When there are complaints about the air quality, building engineers measure carbon dioxide levels to assess the ventilation. But the standard for ventilation is based only on human comfort; there is no built-in consideration for chemical contamination.

A review of the peer-reviewed literature published from 1995 to 2010 found 77 studies that measured chemical pollutants in residences in the United States and in countries with similar lifestyles. The review considered all chemical contaminants measured in the residential indoor air. There were 267 different pollutants found. Chronic-exposure health standards were available for only 97 of the 267 pollutants. Of those 97 pollutants:

- ☐ 15 exceeded the standards in a large fraction of homes
- ☐ nine other pollutants were identified as potential chronic health hazards in a substantial minority of homes
- ☐ an additional nine were identified as potential hazards in only a very small percentage of homes
- ☐ the remaining 64 percent — potentially found in your house — had no health standards.

No studies have been done on potential adverse health impacts from additive or synergistic effects.

Compounds in Indoor Air

New or renovated buildings have higher VOC concentrations. The canaries — patients who claimed to be sensitive to chemicals — had already described these chemical pollutant sources in the 1980s. They identified them by their adverse reactions to various chemical sources indoors that appeared to be tolerated by others. The environmentally sensitive patients usually obtained relief by going outside. Those with sick building syndrome could not identify the individual pollutants responsible for their symptoms, but they still obtained relief by leaving that particular environment. All of us experience these exposures, but most of us are not aware of any health effects.

Here is a list of exposures known to trigger symptoms in patients with multiple chemical sensitivities. The common denominator is that they are all sources of VOCs.

Air freshener	Garage fumes	Paint thinner
Aftershave lotion	Glass cleaner	Perfume
Asphalt fumes	Gasoline products	Pesticides
Carpet (new)	Glue	Rubber
Cologne	Hair spray/gel	Shampoo
Cosmetics (scented)	Insect repellent	Silver polish
Deodorant	Laundry detergent	Skin lotions (scented)
Deodorizers	Magazine scent strips	Soap
Detergent	Marking pens	Tar fumes
Diesel exhaust	Mothballs	Tile cleaner
Dry cleaning solvents	Nail polish	Tobacco smoke
Fabric softener	Nail polish remover	Varnish
Floor cleaner	Newsprint	Vehicle exhaust
Furniture polish	Paint	Vinyl

Because of the difficulty and expense of identifying the individual VOCs in any given building, commercially available assessments measure only the total amount of VOCs, called TVOCs. However, there are many other chemical pollutant exposures that are not accounted for.

Another group of organic chemicals are those that off-gas much more slowly and tend to exist in a more solid phase. These are the semi-volatile organic compounds (SVOCs). They exist as major additives in materials such as floor coverings, furnishings, and electronic components, as well as the active ingredients in pesticides, cleaning agents, and personal care products. The production of SVOCs has increased within the past half-century or so because of their extensive use in commercial products; many SVOCs are commonly more abundant indoors than outside. Of major importance is the fact that the techniques used to capture TVOCs in indoor air quality studies do not capture or measure the SVOCs.

SVOCs tend to be attracted to and accumulate on the surfaces of solids. As a result, they are found in the dust in our homes. SVOCs hang around and can persist indoors for years because of their tendency to bounce back and forth between gas and solid phases. Indoor persistent SVOCs and outdoor persistent organic pollutants (POPs) have a lot in common. Overall, exposures can occur via inhalation, ingestion, or skin contact pathways. Skin and incidental ingestion depend on the concentrations of SVOCs on surfaces that we come into contact with.

The CDC and Health Canada studies that measured and tracked the body burden of pollutants revealed measurable levels of more than a hundred SVOCs, and for some of those compounds the average body burden increased from one survey to the next. SVOCs include flame retardants, plasticizers, and lubricants and are found in a wide range of products. For decades we have employed flame-retardant chemical additives to reduce the flammability of resins and polymers found in commercial products such as furniture, mattresses, electronics (e.g., computers, televisions, cellphones), and even children's products such as car seats, strollers, crib mattresses, and baby clothing. Flame retardants have been shown to leach or otherwise escape from these products over time and accumulate in both the indoor and outdoor environments. Many of the chemical ingredients in flame-retardant mixtures are proprietary and are thus not disclosed by the manufacturers, even to manufacturers who use these chemicals in their final end products (e.g., furniture).

Just like outdoor air, indoor air is also contaminated with particulate matter (PM). Generally there is less indoors than outside because of the filtration effect of the building, but contributions from indoor sources make the PM contents different from those outside. Natural sources of indoor particulates include soil tracked in by shoes, human skin, animal dander from pets, dust mite droppings, particles from other insects, moulds, and bacteria. When enough particulate matter accumulates to become visible, we recognize it as dust. Human activities such as cooking, especially with gas appliances, burning candles, food particles, and especially tobacco smoke are all sources of particulate matter. VOCs are sources of PM, and the quality of indoor PM is especially influenced by absorption of SVOCs, so indoor PM frequently contains plastics, fire retardants, and even pesticides if used locally.

The Inside Story

In June 2011 the journal *Indoor Air* celebrated its 20th anniversary, and one of the articles was a review of the published research on indoor air during those 20 years. It was heartening to note that while fewer than 60 papers were published in indoor chemistry research from 1991 to 2000, in the years from 2001 to 2010 the number almost quadrupled, to 210. It is now recognized that indoor air has become a significant health problem.

We see outdoor air pollution as a dynamic system, constantly in flux. The quality and accumulation of pollutants in the atmosphere are constantly changing, driven largely by complex weather changes and the effects of heat and sunlight. The indoor environment was considered a static box in which physical and chemical transformations of air pollutants were absent or negligible. The usual approaches to understanding indoor air pollution considered only the source of the pollutant: how much was being emitted and for how long, and how much was diluted by ventilation. The fact that primary chemicals from different sources can mix with each other to make new, secondary pollutants was not considered. Neither was the fact that some outdoor air pollution makes its way indoors to compound the problem.

Because of this major oversight, our estimates for primary indoor air pollutant concentrations were low and the secondary pollutants produced were being ignored. Now we know that the concentration of pollutants in indoor air is a function of many factors, including outdoor pollution concentration, indoor sources, ventilation, mixing of these substances, and the chemical reactions occurring between the various pollutants.

The Breathing Zone

Indoor air is a dynamic system, constantly in flux, even in your house, right where you are presently sitting, reading this book. You can't see it or feel it, but it is constantly happening on your skin and on the mucous membranes covering your eyes and respiratory tract. You too are part of this dynamic system. Your immune system is responding — hopefully doing a good job filtering and removing these substances without over-reacting. Some of the pollutants are being exhaled; some are not moving, remaining where they have been deposited on the walls of your respira-tory tract; and others are being absorbed into your body. Some will be stored in various tissues while others are being degraded, detoxified, and eliminated.

We are finally recognizing the contributions of chemicals that are applied to our body and clothing to the breathing zone. These chemical sources from our personal activities form a cloud around our bodies that has not been considered in the past when measuring human exposures.

We used to think that chemicals in the indoor air were stable, part-ly because the technology used could not detect the by-products of the chemical processes that were occurring. However, chemicals in indoor air can — and frequently do — react with one another, either in the gas phase or on surfaces. This incessant dynamic process, known as indoor chemistry, continuously changes the type and concentration of chemicals present in indoor environments.

Ozone in Your House

The indoor chemical reactions that have been studied the most involve ozone, and the most prominent source of indoor ozone is outdoor air. Although there is less ozone indoors because the building acts as a filter, indoor levels still range from 30 to 70 percent of outdoor levels, and they rise and fall according to the levels outside. Ozone tends to react easily with other chemicals to form new and potentially more toxic pollutants.

The recent emphasis on natural or "green" cleaning products has led to an increase in the use of naturally derived chemicals called terpenes, which come from the essential oils of many plants. Examples of terpenes frequently found in cleaners and air fresheners include alpha-pinene, limonene, and delta-carene. You can now make your house, office, or car smell like a pine forest, citrus, various exotic fruits, flowers, vanilla, or cinnamon. These terpenes may be derived from natural sources, but it is not natural to be constantly exposed to high levels of them indoors, especially because they react with other pollutants in the indoor environment, particularly ozone, to form new chemicals. The increased use of terpenes as odorants and cleaning products, together with higher ozone levels indoors plus reduced ventilation, has contributed significantly to our exposures to toxic chemicals.

Fragrances and IAQ

When you read product labels, remember that there is no exact definition for *scent-free*, *fragrance-free*, or *unscented*. The terms *fragrance-free* and *unscented* may mean that no fragrances have been added to the product, but they could also mean that another chemical, called a masking agent, is hiding the scents of the other ingredients in the product.

Speaking of fragrances, it's not just cleaners and deodorizers that pollute the indoor environment. Of greater concern are perfumes and cosmetics, which increase personal chemical exposure for the wearer. Both reactive terpenes and ozone are present in the personal breathing zone of someone who is wearing fragrances. Depending on the product, increases as high as 200 percent in ultrafine particles can be found in the wearer's breathing zone, even 20 to 30 minutes after application of perfume or hairspray. These products are also absorbed through the skin. Furthermore, there is a negative effect on overall indoor air quality for everyone in the room.

VOCs are responsible for the fragrance of scented products. More than 50 different VOCs have been identified in products such as perfumes, deodorants, moisturizers, soaps, fabric softeners, and air fresheners. Fragranced products generate potentially substantial levels of VOCs as well as ultrafine particles in the indoor environment, especially when mixed with ozone. Exposure to these chemicals indoors is associated with risk for developing airway and eye irritations, asthma, and multiple allergic diseases, especially in children. Fragranced consumer products are also associated with headaches, especially migraines. More than 40 percent of people with migraines report perfume as a trigger.

In two surveys of more than 2,100 people, 30.5 percent of the general population reported that they found scented products on others irritating. In addition, 19 percent reported adverse health effects from air fresheners, with higher percentages among those who had asthma and chemical sensitivity.

Industrial-Strength Fragrances

Researchers did a study to identify VOCs emitted from 25 widely used fragranced consumer products. In its market category each of the 25 products was ranked in the top five in annual U.S. sales, and more than half were the top-selling brand. The study reported that 19 of the 25 products had made some claim about being "green" or used a related word in their advertising. The study categorized the products as follows:

- ☐ four laundry products (detergents, dryer sheets, and fabric softener)
- ☐ nine personal care products (soaps, hand sanitizer, lotions, deodorant, shampoo, and baby shampoo)
- ☐ four cleaning supplies (household and industrial cleaning supplies, disinfectants, and dish detergent)
- ☐ eight air fresheners (sprays, gels, solids, and deodorant disks).

The researchers identified 133 VOCs and found that 24 were classified as toxic or hazardous under at least one federal U.S. law. Each product emitted between one and eight of these chemicals. Of the 19 most frequently occurring chemicals in the products, five were classified as toxic or hazardous. The perfume industry would argue that the levels of exposure were low; however, 11 of the products emitted one or more carcinogenic hazardous air pollutants, which have no safe threshold of exposure, according to the EPA.

The Environmental Working Group (EWG), which produced the study of pollutants in cord blood, also did a study of 17 personal care products. It was not published in a peer-reviewed journal but is available online. Of the 17 products tested, 13 were purchased in the United States and four in Canada. The EWG found 91 different ingredients. It stated that the Cosmetic Ingredient Review, an industry-funded self-policing body, had assessed only 19 of the 91 ingredients, and that the International Fragrance Association and the Research Institute for Fragrance Materials, which develop and set voluntary standards for chemicals in the "fragrance" component of products, had assessed only 27 of the 91 ingredients. The EWG reported average findings per product as follows:

- ☐ 29 chemical ingredients per label
- ☐ 14 secret chemicals (found in the testing but not on the label)
- ☐ 10 sensitizing chemicals (which can trigger allergic reactions)
- ☐ 4 hormone disruptors (which can disrupt natural hormones)
- ☐ 12 chemicals that had never been assessed for safety by government or industry.

The fragrance industry argues that it follows proper protocols for testing its products. But you won't find those studies published in peer-reviewed medical journals because law protects the industry from disclosing the nature of its ingredients, citing proprietary reasons. Even personal care products are not required to list the ingredients used in fragrances.

Surface Chemistry

What all this means is that indoor air is a soup, and the recipe calls for constantly adding chemicals while stirring continuously. The contents are particulate matter, VOCs, SVOCs, other chemicals, ozone, and biological substances such as mould. These contents are constantly being mixed in the air, their interactions produce new and different particulate matter, and a process known as oxidation (which will be examined later) occurs upon contact with ozone to produce different chemicals.

There is a process known as surface chemistry. If you ever participated in experiments in the chemistry lab, you used a little heater called a Bunsen burner. Heat brings chemicals together at a rapid rate and therefore speeds up chemical reactions, bringing them together to form new compounds. The larger the surface area, the more chemicals are attracted to it to mix with others, which accelerates the process, increasing the speed of reactions of pollutants by as much as 10 to 100 times. Ozone, which comes in from the outside, contributes to this process.

There is more surface area indoors (compared to outdoors), where these chemical reactions are occurring. These surfaces include walls, floors (especially carpets), furniture, and all the objects inside your home. Your body is a surface as well. Chemical reactions are constantly taking place on your skin and eyes, in your nose and throat, and on the linings of your bronchial tubes. These reactions add to indoor air pollution, especially in your personal breathing zone. Scientists are just beginning to understand that measuring a person's exposures is different from simply checking pollution in the indoor air. When human surfaces are complicated by the addition of chemical compounds such as perfumes and soaps, ozone attracted to those surfaces mixes with the chemicals to form new products that may be even more toxic.

Assessing Indoor Air

Because of this constantly changing chemical soup, the quantity of total VOCs (TVOCs) does not have much significance. Furthermore, these measurements should not be used to determine the intensity or acceptability of chemical exposures indoors because they do not describe which individual chemicals are present. Unfortunately, when building engineers assess IAQ in response to complaints by people in the building, usually the only way they assess pollution levels is by measuring TVOCs. Building owners or management frequently dismiss complaints; they assume that there are no problems with the indoor environment because the TVOC levels are considered "normal."

Logic suggests that all these daily chemical exposures must be burdening our detoxification systems. Are the patients with sick building syndrome and multiple chemical sensitivities really canaries? Can they sense these chemical exposures better than the rest of the population? What about the rest of us? Are we at risk? Should we be more cautious and reduce our exposures?

It starts with the choices we make regarding products we use in the home and the workplace, what we apply to our bodies, and how well we ventilate. When we paint or renovate, we can choose safer materials. We can use paints that don't emit VOCs. We can keep the windows open and sleep somewhere else. We can let materials such as new furniture and mattresses off-gas before bringing them into the home.

In Canada and some U.S. states the building code now requires an air exchanger to assist in ventilation (older homes are grandfathered). Indoor air is more contaminated than outdoor air. If your house doesn't have an air exchanger, it should be a priority to install one with a high-efficiency particulate air (HEPA) filter. This is the best filter system to reduce particulate matter in your home.

Driving in Hazardous Conditions

The indoor environment also includes transportation: depending on where we live, we spend almost six percent of a typical day inside a vehicle. For many people in big cities, a relatively large proportion of daily exposure to a multitude of pollutants occurs while commuting. Compared to the air outside, exposure to pollution from the outdoors (especially particulate matter) is higher in cars, and it is highest in diesel buses. One reason is the resuspension of particulate matter caused by traffic movement. The faster the traffic, the greater the number of particles resuspended. Not surprisingly, particulate matter exposures are lowest in electric buses and streetcars. Particulate matter in underground subway stations is generally higher than on the street, as subways generate their own particles from wheel–rail contact and braking.

Airflow into a vehicle increases when you go faster, and the amount of increase in airflow is greater in older vehicles because they are less airtight. When we use the recirculation damper, we reduce exposure to pollutants from outside but increase exposure to those generated from materials inside the vehicle, although older cars will have off-gassed more than new ones.

Are these daily exposures significant? In a small study, nine North Carolina Highway Patrol troopers (aged 23 to 30) were monitored on four successive days. Their increased exposure to particulate matter reduced heart rate variability, a change that identifies patients with an increased risk of cardiac mortality. A similar finding has been reported in a small study of taxi drivers. Although larger studies may possibly prove them to be irrelevant, these findings are certainly not surprising, given the observed increased particulate matter in vehicles and the well-documented relationship of levels of particulate matter with risk for heart disease.

At home or at work, and even on the way to work, we are in an indoor environment. The air that we breathe is the largest source of pollutant assaults that our bodies have to deal with. We were all born with natural detoxification systems, but they weren't intended to deal with the chemical soup that we live in today. Chronic illnesses are on the rise, and new conditions such as chronic fatigue syndrome, fibromyalgia, and multiple chemical sensitivities have emerged. The fact that the increase in our chemical exposures occurred at the same time as the change in health patterns raises the suspicion that these phenomena are linked. The MCS canaries are trying to tell us that there is indeed a cause-and-effect relationship.

CHAPTER 7

HOW OUR BODIES COPE

Sit down before Mother Nature as a small child. Be prepared to cast aside all preconceived notions and to follow her into whatever abyss she leads, or you shall learn nothing.

— Thomas Huxley

For more than 30 years I have witnessed a constant stream of new patients with the symptoms of chronic fatigue syndrome (CFS), fibromyalgia, and multiple chemical sensitivities (MCS). But because there are no biological markers that can point to malfunction in a particular tissue or organ, many doctors automatically assume that the illness is not real, that these patients cannot be suffering from a medical condition, that they are all mentally ill and in denial. That conclusion is based on deduction: if it is not physical, it must be mental. Since the premise of this book is that the polluted environment causes these conditions, that these patients are biologically ill, and that they are canaries warning us of the dangers of pollution exposures, where is the science to support it? Where are the biological clues?

The process of developing a chronic illness begins long before it can be detected clinically. If we can understand the processes, maybe that can help explain the link with pollution exposures. In order to do so, we need to look more closely, deeper inside the body, to see how the cells handle the onslaught of manmade molecules that we refer to as xenobiotics, and what happens if they can't handle the load.

Cell Civilization

Cells can perform all the basic functions of life independently: they absorb oxygen and food, convert it to energy, eliminate waste products, and reproduce. They are the smallest unit of life — nothing else smaller is capable of surviving on its own. We can survive on our own too. However, I know that would be really difficult for me. I am not a talented hunter-gatherer, so I depend on others to supply my food and provide electricity for my home. In fact, we are all specialists of some sort and depend on other members of our civilization to survive. The human body contains three trillion cells. They may be capable of independent living but they are also specialized and need each other for survival. Our body is a civilization made up of cells.

The cell is a living sac of a gel-like fluid called cytoplasm that is supported by proteins and surrounded by a membrane. Floating around inside the cytoplasm are structures called organelles, which have specific functions that contribute to the cell's metabolism. Organelles are the cells' version of organs. The term *metabolism* is used to describe all the physical and chemical processes that take place within a living organism. Cell metabolism produces by-products that need to be broken down and eliminated.

Mitochondria

Mitochondria are organelles that play a critical role in energy metabolism. They are vitally involved in whether a cell lives or dies, because they create and store fuel for the cell's activities. They use oxygen and food nutrients to generate and then store energy for the cell to use. There are hundreds or even thousands of mitochondria in every animal cell, with the amount depending on how active that cell is supposed to be.

Mitochondria were once free-living bacteria with a special talent for producing energy. Larger cells engulfed them, taking them into their cytoplasm, planning to digest them for food. But because they profited from the extra energy provided, they postponed digesting this extra energy source. These cells were able to survive longer and thus evolved to live in a symbiotic relationship with the power-producing bacteria they had engulfed. After millions of years the mitochondria are now part of the structure of modern cells.

There is interesting evidence to support this theory. First of all, mitochondria have their own DNA. Second, they cannot be generated *de novo*; that is, they cannot be constructed or created by the cell. They can be derived only from preexisting mitochondria, which proliferate by division into two, like a cell. This process is known as mitochondrial biogenesis. They also move about in the cell and frequently fuse to mix and unify their contents to maintain good quality control. All these processes have important consequences for cell life and death.

After cells divide in two, each new cell begins its own life cycle. At first mitochondria reproduce to supply more energy so that the cell can make more organelles and perform its function well. Eventually the cell becomes ready to divide again. Once again biogenesis of the mitochondria is essential to meet the cell's increased energy demands required for division. If there are not enough healthy mitochondria at the beginning, the cell never gets to function properly. If there are not enough mitochondria in the preparation stage, cell division cannot occur. Because aging decreases the number and functioning of mitochondria, there is less cell regeneration as we grow older.

About 98 percent of the oxygen we inhale is consumed by mitochondria. Our requirement for oxygen in order to stay alive is based on the mitochondrial demand for it. They use the oxygen and nutrients from food, such as glucose, to generate packets of energy called adenosine triphosphate (ATP), which they can also easily store, transfer, and transform to release and provide energy when required. Mitochondria are the source of energy, strength, and vitality for every cell. As the powerhouse of cells, they provide energy for everything the cell needs to do. Hundreds or thousands of well-functioning mitochondria travel around each cell, distributing the readily available energy from the ATP they have produced to wherever it is needed. Metabolically, this is where the action is inside a cell. The by-products of this metabolism are toxic waste products that need to be destroyed or eliminated. Unfortunately, the mitochondria sit in the middle of it all.

Mitochondria and Oxygen

Oxygen itself is toxic. That may come as a surprise, because we usually think of oxygen as pure, vital, or even healing. But oxygen, if not processed properly, is poisonous.

Millions of years ago, when plants came into being, they produced lots of oxygen and changed the atmosphere. Cells had to adapt to their increased exposure to oxygen. It was the mitochondria that learned to convert toxic oxygen into energy; as the evolutionary story goes, some cells then incorporated mitochondria internally. However, the by-products of this energy production and increased metabolism are toxic and can cause damage.

To survive, the cells had to quickly learn to break down and eliminate those toxic by-products, a skill that has evolved into our detoxification system. It is a sophisticated and efficient system that has been present in every complex evolved cell for many millions of years, but it was not designed to cope with the quantity and variety of pollutants we have been taking into our bodies since the Second World War.

Free radicals are *the enemy within.* They are the waste products of the cell's metabolism. They are produced in small amounts under normal physiological conditions, by essential metabolic processes. When a cell increases its metabolism because it is required to work extra hard, free radical production is also increased.

Free radicals cause damage. They will rip an electron from the nearest molecule, which in turn does so to a neighbouring molecule, starting a chain reaction. They operate like vampires, which change their victims into vampires too after they steal their blood. This snowball effect can wreak havoc on cells, causing damage that may eventually reduce cell function and even contribute to cell death. However, the cell has a system to stop this chain reaction and detoxify the toxic molecules. It uses antioxidants, which can neutralize free radicals and stop the chain reaction of damage.

Detoxification: Phase 1 and 2 Biotransformation

Every cell is naturally equipped with a detoxification system. Waste that cannot be completely degraded must be detoxified and eliminated from the body. The liver is one of the specialist organs for detoxification, and it can also discharge toxins into the gastrointestinal system via bile. The body excretes toxins via the kidneys, the gastrointestinal system, and, to a lesser degree, perspiration.

Many xenobiotics are highly lipophilic, meaning that they dissolve in or attach to oil or fat. As a result they can accumulate in the brain, which is rich in oils, but most are stored in visceral fat, the fat inside your belly. Because they are not water-soluble, they are hard to excrete and require a structural alteration — called biotransformation — to get rid of them, or else they will remain in the body for a long time. Fortunately, a multitude of enzyme systems exist in every cell, especially in the liver, that are uniquely capable of converting fat-soluble substances into more water-soluble derivatives, which can then be more efficiently excreted by the kidneys or even our sweat and breath.

Biotransformation is a process that is studied extensively by drug companies. It is important to know how, and how quickly, the body breaks down pharmaceuticals. Pharmacists warn us to be careful when we use two medications together if they use the same detoxification system. If the medications are broken down and eliminated more slowly than usual because they have to share that system, the prescribed doses of both could be too high.

The breakdown of drugs and chemicals takes many steps to complete. Along that pathway of detoxification, new and different chemical structures are produced, and they may also have the potential to be active or toxic.

There are two phases in biotransformation. The Phase 1 enzyme system prepares the original substance through various mechanisms so that it is capable of being connected with or added on to another substance. This connection occurs in Phase 2 of the pathway and makes the compound water-soluble and thus easier to excrete. The two phases must work at the same speed. If Phase 1 is much faster than Phase 2, the new activated substances formed by Phase 1 will accumulate, often with potential to cause damage. There is a buildup of intermediary metabolites, which are usually free radicals, or toxic by-products.

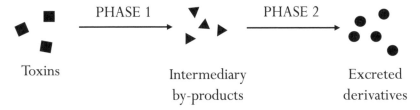

<table>
<tr><td>Toxins</td><td>PHASE 1 →
Intermediary
by-products</td><td>PHASE 2 →
Excreted
derivatives</td></tr>
</table>

If this system does not function efficiently or is overwhelmed, there can be a buildup of the original substance and/or its active intermediary by-products, which in some cases can be more toxic than the parent. For example, acetaminophen (Tylenol) is the most widely used pharmaceutical analgesic (pain-reducing) and antipyretic (fever-reducing) agent in the world; it is found in more than 100 products. As such it is one of the most common pharmaceuticals associated with both intentional and unintentional poisoning. Acetaminophen toxicity is caused by the inability of the Phase 2 detoxification system to keep pace with Phase 1. As a result, significant liver damage can be caused by accumulation of a toxic intermediary by-product once the liver's antioxidant stores are depleted. The antidote is an antioxidant, N-acetylcysteine.

For the efficient and successful operation of both Phase 1 and Phase 2 biotransformation pathways, it is also essential that all the nutrients required for their function be available in adequate amounts.

This detoxification system, which evolved on a cellular and organ level over millions of years, is now being asked to help clear out increasingly more xenobiotics, daily and simultaneously. While some of these chemicals do have short half-lives and can be easily eliminated from our bodies, we are incapable of maintaining their absence, because our exposure to them is so frequent. One example is bisphenol A (BPA), a chemical found in hard plastics and the coatings of food and drink cans. Add this problem to the load of other xenobiotics that have longer half-lives or are persistent and cannot be eliminated for years, and the potential for overburdening our detoxification systems increases.

Those who insist that the traditional toxicology paradigm is absolute will argue that our usual exposures to these various chemical pollutants are not toxic. But does everyone's detoxification system have the same capability to handle the total load? What would happen if one or both phases of the detoxification system could not keep up with the daily demands placed on them by our constant and unintended intake of xenobiotics? What is their potential to influence our chances of morbidity or mortality?

Failure of Detoxification and Oxidative Stress

Oxidative stress is the term used to describe the imbalance between the production of oxidants or other free radicals and our ability to neutralize or detoxify them. It refers to any of the pathologic changes seen in living cells that occur in response to excessive levels of these toxic molecules. In research labs we can observe the imbalance by measuring the levels of oxidants or free radicals, or we can assume that it is occurring when we find low levels of antioxidants.

We know that oxidative stress is occurring when we find evidence of damage and destruction inside cells. Oxidative stress damages DNA, especially mitochondrial DNA, as well as lipids in cell and organelle membranes, and various proteins. We can measure the resulting by-products of this damage in blood or urine.

Oxidative stress and DNA damage can cause significant changes in cell function. The mitochondria are most likely to be damaged, not only because they produce free radicals as waste products but also because they are immersed in them, making them highly vulnerable to attack. If damaged, their functional ability to produce energy efficiently is re-duced. By stimulating cell activity and measuring the levels of substances normally used by working mitochondria, we can assess mitochondrial function. These substances get used up when the mitochondria are more active. If they aren't functioning well, the levels of the substances will remain the same.

A reduction in the number and functioning of mitochondria will eventually have an adverse effect on cell function. The cell relies on en-ergy supplied by the mitochondria. A plethora of studies show that free radicals and mitochondrial DNA mutations are associated with cellular injury, aging mechanisms, and accumulated toxicity. If enough mito-chondria are damaged, the cell will actually give up and program itself for a tidy, well-planned suicide. This is known as apoptosis. Needless to say, if enough cells in a tissue die, the result is organ malfunction or degeneration.

All humans have hundreds of chemical pollutants stored in their bodies and daily exposure to many others, all of which impose demands on the detoxification systems of all cells. This chemical burden has built up in every human, including our unborn children, within the past 60 years — in just over two generations. Given that the detoxification sys-tems evolved over millions of years, how capable are they of handling the recent, continually rising challenge of chemical accumulation? Are these exposures significant? What happens if we get oxidatively stressed out?

Environmental chemical exposures in urban populations are asso-ciated with oxidative stress because production of oxidants is one of the body's responses to the constant chemical burden. These exposures appear to be causing oxidative stress-related disorders, regardless of the types of chemicals involved. Clearly, all the chemicals we have introduced into our personal environments have the potential to cause oxidative stress in the body, as our biological systems have not had adequate time to adapt to the rapidly changing chemical environment.

An increase in oxidants does not necessarily cause oxidative stress if it can be counterbalanced by our cellular antioxidant network. But the relentless exposure to environmental chemicals, combined with lifestyle factors such as smoking, unhealthy diet, and physical inactivity, as well as certain genetic factors, may be contributing to increased oxidative stress. On the other hand, cutting down our intake of pollutants will diminish the burden on our detoxification systems and reduce the oxidative stress effect.

Indoor Pollution and Oxidative Stress

Oxidative stress has been found in industrial workers who were exposed to VOCs. It could be argued that their exposures were higher than an average person's. However, oxidative stress has also been demonstrated in non-industrial office workers with sick building syndrome, even though the IAQ was considered "normal."

Oxidative stress is a mechanism that contributes to the adverse health effects of air pollutant exposures. Many published papers have demonstrated, both in living organisms and in test-tube studies, that oxidative stress results from exposure to chemicals such as polyaromatic hydrocarbons (PAHs), VOCs, BPA, or plasticizers. Oxidative stress is part of the normal process of aging, but now a considerable contribution is coming from pollutants.

Patients with multiple chemical sensitivities (MCS) are more likely to have an abnormal genotype for the enzyme systems of detoxification, which makes them more likely to develop oxidative stress. But even MCS patients with normal detoxification genotypes demonstrate significant oxidative stress. How is oxidative stress related to chemical sensitivities? If the relationship is significant, oxidative stress must be contributing to the mechanism of MCS. That would justify and verify the claim that MCS patients are canaries, warning those who are not so sensitive that they are in danger too.

PART III

ENVIRONMENTAL ILLNESS

CHAPTER 8

MCS EXISTS

The hardest thing to explain is the glaringly evident which everybody has decided not to see.

— Ayn Rand, *The Fountainhead*

Many people argue that multiple chemical sensitivities (MCS) does not exist, that patients are falsely attributing their symptoms to pollutant exposures. According to the traditional toxicology and immunology paradigms, chemical sensitivity does not make sense. There is no evidence to support any biological phenomenon explaining the reactions. If evidence can be found, then the traditional paradigms are wrong.

C.L. is a 44-year-old woman who came to see me because of a sensitivity to the odours of chemicals. Her symptoms had lasted one and a half years. When she was exposed to various chemical scents, symptoms were provoked, including cough, mental fatigue, nausea, and headache. Triggering scents included perfumes and other scented products, such as soaps, detergents, fabric softeners, cleaners, and deodorizers, as well as diesel, newsprint, fresh paint, and plastics. If she removed herself from the odour immediately, the symptoms would abate slowly. Sometimes they were gone after half an hour; sometimes they lasted the rest of the day. C.L. also reported that, since the onset of her sensitivities, she seemed to have a more acute sense of smell than other people.

C.L.'s environmental exposure history revealed that she was worse at work; when she was at home or in other venues where those odours could be avoided, she had no symptoms. She worked in a downtown high-rise office building at an overpass above a major roadway, and there was also an underground garage beneath the building complex. Prior to the onset of her illness there was evidence of problems with the quality of the indoor air. She and her colleagues could frequently smell odours from the traffic below, which they attributed to buses idling right outside the building. Furthermore, they could often smell the odour from diesel generators used during construction in the underground parking garage.

Consultation with an allergist confirmed that C.L. had allergies to ragweed and penicillin, which she had had since childhood, but ruled out allergies as a cause for her present symptoms. A consultation with a respirologist had ruled out asthma or other lung conditions as a cause for her cough. She had no symptoms of anxiety or depression and there were no psychosocial stressors, either recently or in her past, to suggest the possibility of psychiatric illness. She also had a long-standing history of gastrointestinal complaints, including heartburn, intestinal flatulence, loose stools, and bloating, and had been diagnosed previously with reflux and irritable bowel syndrome (IBS).

C.L.'s illness pattern is consistent with the case criteria for sick building syndrome (SBS) and multiple chemical sensitivities. The environment of the workplace can provoke symptoms. She reacts to odours previously tolerated and tolerated by others. She has multiple system complaints: brain, respiratory, and gastrointestinal. She also has a history of allergies, IBS, and reflux, all of which are frequently co-morbid with MCS; that is, these syndromes are more likely to occur together.

The only known treatment for this disorder is avoidance of triggers — in other words, environmental control. Being allowed to work from home was the eventual accommodation. Once this was successfully initiated, she enjoyed a normal lifestyle as long as she was able to avoid chemical scents. She gradually became somewhat less sensitive, such that the onset of symptoms was not so rapid. If she experienced an exposure, such as to a perfumed product, she could move away immediately and symptoms would not be provoked.

What happened to C.L.? Although several colleagues had complained when the air quality at work was poor because they had also been exposed to the same pollutants, none of them developed multiple chemical sensitivities. If she is simply phobic about chemicals, why doesn't she have other symptoms of anxiety? Why did C.L. become a canary?

What has made MCS controversial is that these patients appear to respond to exposures to chemicals they used to tolerate and that are tolerated by everyone else, and their symptoms are provoked by levels that are not considered toxic. Even stranger is the fact that they react to different substances that are chemically unrelated. Can the brain really become sensitive to multiple different chemicals, or is it stress? Is MCS physical or mental? The answer to all these questions is yes.

The contentious assertion that MCS exists in the patients' heads may actually be the common ground where finally the dispute may be ended. Sensitization to chemicals in MCS is a brain disorder; the medical argument is one of causation. Those who resist the concept that reactions to low-dose chemicals could be physiologically induced are using reductionist reasoning. They conclude that because the patients have no biological abnormalities and the symptom-triggering chemical exposures are not toxic, the cause of MCS must be a psychiatric abnormality and the symptoms must be stress related. An alternative explanation is that the stress response is triggered by chemical exposures, that the triggering doses are not toxic but the brain reacts because it has become chemically sensitized, and that the process of sensitization is initiated by oxidative stress. Let's examine the medical evidence to see what is actually happening in MCS patients' heads.

The Limbic System

The human brain is large and complex and — more than any other of our attributes — it defines us as humans. The part of the brain that separates us most from all the other animals is the cortex. Ours is so big that to accommodate the size it is folded up like an accordion, so that when we look at pictures of the human brain, what we see are numerous folds and grooves. Not only is our cortex the largest, it also has the densest and most complex neuron interconnections, which enable us to perform our unique human activities. The cortex is responsible for auditory perception, language, memory, visual information processing, voluntary movement, spatial orientation, touch interpretation, and number processing. It is especially important because it is involved in emotions, problem solving, critical thinking, the ability to plan, and recognition of parts of speech.

The brain of primitive animals, such as reptiles, contains a cerebellum to control movement and a brainstem. The brainstem is the smallest part of the brain and sits at the top of the spinal cord. Its job is to keep us alive. It controls our heart rate and makes our lungs breathe. Breaking your neck can result in death because of damage to the brainstem. The evolutionary gap between the reptilian brain and our highly developed cortex is bridged by the limbic system. The limbic system is where the biological response to stress takes place. When animals, including humans, are confronted by a perceived stressor, we become ready to fight or to run. This is known as the fight-or-flight phenomenon.

The purpose of the limbic system is survival and adaptation to the environment. To do its job, this system communicates with the environment using all the senses, including sight, hearing, touch, smell, and taste, as well as with the immune system. Birds know to fly south in the winter because they sense fewer hours of sunlight. There is bidirectional communication with all the other systems in the brain, including the cortex and the sensory and hormone control systems. This communication also extends to other systems in the body, such as the gastrointestinal system and the immune system, which is constantly scanning the external environment.

Fear, hunger, and thirst are the basic motivators for self-preservation in all animals, including humans. We have all experienced fear and the stress response it provokes. Any stimulus, whether from the external environment or the internal milieu, results in several adaptive reactions to meet the needs of the organism, all regulated through limbic pathways. These include emotional, autonomic, motor, and cognitive responses linked to memory and motivation, which are other major functions of the limbic system. A simplified but accurate view is that the whole system is geared to recognition of and reaction to new stimuli.

Imagine sitting, quietly reading at home, when suddenly there is a sound of breaking glass behind you. Within hundredths of a second, the auditory (hearing) nerve sends a signal to the hippocampus, a part of the limbic system, which immediately compares this noise to all the stored previous experiences (memory). At the same time, the hypothalamus is stimulated to trigger a stress response. Your heart rate and blood pressure increase and you start sweating. Meanwhile, the hippocampus realizes that this surprising noise cannot be explained, and it tells the amygdala, another part of the limbic system, to generate the emotion of fear. This prompts you to action.

The amygdala simultaneously sends messages to other parts of your brain, causing you to quickly turn towards the source of the sound to see what's happening. At this point the cortex analyzes the visual and auditory information and responds back to the limbic system. The response of fear and stress will increase if you see a stranger who has just invaded your home through a broken window, or it will shut down if it is just the family cat that has knocked over your glass of wine.

The limbic system influences or is influenced by aggression and fear, pleasure, reward and addiction, and sexuality. It is involved in:

- ☐ cognition
- ☐ mood and emotion
- ☐ autonomic nervous system function
- ☐ attention processing
- ☐ decision making
- ☐ short-term memory

- storage in long-term memory
- spatial memory
- the sleep/wake cycle
- pain
- immune function.

The limbic system reads cues from the environment, both external and internal, and tries to maintain balance, or homeostasis. It responds to cues. It uses concentration and memory to learn to survive. If a stranger were to threaten you with a gun, you would never forget that person's face; it would be forever memorized as an enemy's. We use our cortex to read the environment. If someone calls you a bitch, you are offended and a stress response is provoked by signals sent to the limbic system — unless you interpret the insult as a joke. If you call your dog a bitch, not only does she not have the cortex to process the information, she couldn't care less.

The cortex is just one source of information about the environment. The limbic system responds to all input from the sensory and immune systems as well. It shares whatever information it receives with all the other systems — all communications are bidirectional. The system works like a conductor and an orchestra. The environment-mind-body connection occurs in this region. If you feel a gentle stroking on your back, it will generate warm and happy feelings if the person responsible is your partner, but you will have a much different response if the perpetrator is a stranger in a crowded subway.

Individuals vary in their sensitivity to stress, whether it is from a physical or an emotional source, because other factors, such as lifestyle, are involved. For example, the strength of the stress response is enhanced by obesity, use of tobacco, and alcohol; it is diminished by exercise. We all know that the more stressed we are by something, the more easily we can be stressed by other factors. This is known as hypervigilance. It is caused by chronic stress, because the initiating hormone for the stress response — called corticotropin-releasing factor — remains elevated, which increases the likelihood of sensitization to other stressors. Thus we feel nervous or anxious or stressed. Hypervigilance is abnormally increased arousal and abnormal awareness of environmental stimuli.

Sensitization and Kindling

Sensitization is the process of becoming susceptible to a given stimulus that previously had no effect or significance. It is the phenomenon that makes us react to something at lower levels than normal, or to something that we shouldn't react to at all. The term *sensitization* has been used in research of brain function in animals for more than 40 years. It is defined as a progressive increase in the size of a response because of repeated stimulations.

In immunology, sensitization is called allergy. In psychology it is the process of becoming highly sensitive to specific emotional events or situations. In MCS it is sensitization of the brain to many chemicals at levels that previously had no relevance. If we understand how sensitization occurs in the brain, we will see the evidence for sensitization to chemicals.

We use kindling in order to get a fire started, and the word also describes a similar occurrence in the brain. Stimulating the brain with electric currents causes seizures. Stimulating the brain for a few weeks at a very low intensity — too low to cause any type of convulsing (seizure or epilepsy) — will eventually cause seizures in rats, even though only very low stimulation is applied. Their brains become sensitized to electricity, and the sensitivity lasts for months.

Chemicals can cause kindling too. Giving rats repeated low doses of chemicals that can induce seizures at higher doses eventually drops the threshold. Giving the rat the previously tolerated low dose then induces a seizure, without any evidence that the chemical has accumulated in the rat. This discovery led researchers to theorize that kindling, as a form of sensitization, provides a plausible biological explanation for the MCS phenomenon. One dissenting argument is that these are only rat studies.

But who would volunteer to have seizures induced by chemicals or electric shock?

There is evidence to support the position that sensitization in the brains of rats can be induced by repeated low-dose exposures to chemicals. Call it kindling or something else, but behavioural or neurochemical alterations in animals can occur from sensitization to various solvents that are normally toxic at higher doses, as well as several different pesticides. Animal experiments also demonstrate that sensitization to one chemical leads to increased sensitivity to other, chemically unrelated substances.

So what if we can turn rats into canaries? Where is the evidence that it can happen to humans? And if it does happen, why doesn't it happen to all of us, since we are all exposed repeatedly to low doses of chemicals? First you need to understand that activating receptors on the cell membranes of neurons induces kindling.

What's a Receptor?

Nerve cells, or neurons, are industrious, energetic, and very highly specialized cells. The term *neuron* is a Greek word for a sinew, string, or wire, and it's an appropriate name for the cells that send and receive electrical signals over long distances. The neuron is an exceptional communicator. It can process and transmit information from one part of the body or brain to another, or to neighbouring neurons, and it does so with amazing speed.

There is an electric charge on the neuron membrane that is passed along from one neuron to the next, as if through a wire. We know how electricity works: the ends of the wires need to touch. On/off power switches connect or disconnect wires, but neuron communication systems are not just the passing on of electric current signals. Neurons don't actually touch each other at all, although their many branches allow them to send signals to different neurons at the same time. To bridge the gap between cells, neurons have developed a chemical messaging system.

Sending a message involves releasing a specific chemical messenger towards a neighbouring neuron. The message will be received if the neuron intended to receive it has the appropriate receptors to capture that chemical messenger. The receptors are situated on the cell membrane and work like a lock and key. Like the space shuttle docking with the space station, the fit must be exact.

These chemical messengers are called neurotransmitters, and they are molecules with different shapes and sizes. Different neurotransmitters can be released and be perceived by the receiving neuron, but only if the neurotransmitter stimulates the right receptor.

Receptors and Oxidative Stress

Oxidative stress causes damage to mitochondria, but damage can occur to other structures as well. One of the molecular structures susceptible to oxidative stress is formed by lipids—fats and oils that play a major role in the structure of the cell membrane. Not only does the cell membrane hold the cell together, it is the interface — the connecting boundary with the external environment. It selects and controls what gets in or out of the cell, and receives communications from neighbouring or distant sources. The cell membrane contains the receptors to receive messages via hormones and neurotransmitters.

Oxidative damage of lipids in cell membranes can damage the membranes and adversely affect the function of receptors. One way the damage does this is by making these receptors, called NMDA receptors, more excitable, which is what happens in kindling. This lends more support to the possibility that oxidative stress could contribute to sensitization in MCS. There are also other receptors on neurons that can be stimulated by oxidative stress. A major one is the TRPV1 receptor, and there is evidence in human studies that these receptors become sensitized in MCS.

TRPV1 Receptors

TRPV1 receptors are also known as capsaicin receptors. Capsaicin is the pungent ingredient in red-hot chili peppers that creates the sensation of heat. To a degree people enjoy the burning sensation from eating peppers, some more than others. Even if you eat a refrigerated hot pepper, the sensation of heat is still created because the capsaicin selectively binds to the receptors known as TRPV1. They reside on the membranes of pain- and heat-sensing neurons in mucous membranes and the skin. When stimulated, these receptors activate neurons to send a message to the brain. Capsaicin is the ingredient in pepper spray, which people use to ward off attacks by dogs, bears, and humans. On contact, pepper spray causes the eyes to burn and the respiratory system to induce coughing.

These capsaicin or TRPV1 receptors are widespread, found in the brain, the eyes, the lining of the bladder, the mast cells of the immune system, the stomach lining, the bowels, the larynx, and the bronchial tubes. Because they are found in the pulmonary system, challenging these receptors with inhalations of capsaicin is used routinely to study coughing.

Capsaicin is a well-known cough-inducing agent. The more sensitive the sensory neurons lining the bronchial tubes, the more easily one can provoke coughing with capsaicin inhalation. Research on cough and cough medicines frequently involves testing with capsaicin-inhalation challenges because it is a reliable testing method. The capsaicin-inhalation challenge test consists of inhaling different concentrations of capsaicin, using a mouthpiece apparatus to control the amount. The total number of coughs provoked is counted over 10 minutes. This test is commonly used in clinical research because it induces coughing in a safe, reliable, dose-dependent, and reproducible manner. Well over a hundred studies using capsaicin-challenge testing have been published.

MCS patients with respiratory symptoms, even without asthma, are hypersensitive to inhalation of capsaicin when compared to controls, and this has been demonstrated by double-blind challenges. Double-blind is an experimental method designed to remove bias, in which neither the test subjects nor the experimenters know if the treatment on trial is real or a placebo (fake). The MCS patients coughed more at lower doses when inhaling capsaicin, and the higher the dose, the more coughs provoked. Other challenge studies have reproduced the same results, demonstrating TRPV1 receptor hypersensitivity in patients with chemical sensitivities.

Clearly patients with MCS have hypersensitive TRPV1 receptors. The hypersensitivity of these receptors explains how and why MCS patients have multiple symptoms from multiple systems. The TRPV1 receptor is especially active in sensory neurons and the brain, notably in the limbic system, where it facilitates long-lasting sensitization. These receptors drive excitation of the neurons to enhance messaging between them.

Many studies show that oxidative stress sensitizes TRPV1 receptors. But although the TRPV1 receptor may be the major target for organic solvents in MCS, it is likely not the only one for chemicals in this illness. Other receptors and mechanisms are probably involved as well. Remember these TRPV1 receptors; I will be referring to them later in the book because they are involved in many chronic conditions besides MCS. Although they didn't know about oxidative stress and sensitization of TRPV1 receptors, the canaries were right to warn us about the dangers of exposures to low doses of chemicals.

Why do some people become sensitized to chemicals more easily than others? The answer is not clear. There are many factors, including genetic susceptibility. Not everyone who smokes gets cancer. There is evidence that MCS patients are genetically predisposed to have inferior enzyme systems for detoxification. Because they are less capable of detoxifying efficiently, oxidative stress occurs more easily, which sensitizes the TRPV1 receptors.

The Blood–Brain Barrier

The brain contains 50 to 100 billion neurons, with as many as 1,000 trillion connections. While it makes up only two percent of the total weight of the body, it uses 25 percent of our basic energy requirements. The brain is the most critical and sensitive organ in the human body, and it requires a highly regulated, secure environment in which to work properly. A barrier, known as the blood–brain barrier, provides this protection.

The blood–brain barrier exists in the lining of the tiniest blood vessels in the brain, the capillaries. They are only one cell thick, to allow contents to pass easily back and forth, in and out of the blood supply. In the brain capillaries, the cells differ from those found elsewhere in the body:

- ☐ They have very tight junctions that provide an effective barrier
- ☐ These tight junctions are held together and regulated by a variety of molecules
- ☐ They are much more restrictive in what they will transport.

The blood–brain barrier plays a crucial role in limiting exposure of the brain to damaging molecules and cells. Because the brain is protected, chemicals should not and cannot get into the brain very easily. So how can they induce sensitization of the limbic system? One way is that if the blood–brain barrier becomes damaged, chemicals can leak in. For example, the barrier can be injured by toxic insult from exposure to heavy metals such as lead, mercury, iron, and manganese, leading to increased permeability and reduced protection. TRPV1 receptors also exist in the blood–brain barrier. Although strong stimulation is required, activation of these receptors can occur, which will cause disruption of the barrier and an increase in permeability.

In one area of the brain (around the third and fourth ventricles) there is no blood–brain barrier, which allows the nervous system to communicate chemically and hormonally with the rest of the body. It allows for crosstalk between the immune, endocrine, and limbic systems. This is an open portal into the brain for the direct entry of chemicals, including medications and street drugs.

There is another way in which chemicals can enter the brain. Several studies, both animal and human, demonstrate that ultrafine particles

(UFPs) can be translocated (transported from one place to another) by the olfactory nerve, which is responsible for the sense of smell, directly into the limbic system. Chemicals that are inhaled and land on the membrane lining of the nasal passages are absorbed directly into the olfactory nerve neurons. They are then carried from one end of the nerve to the other, directly into the brain, bypassing the blood–brain barrier.

The Case for MCS

What had happened to C.L.? She was describing sensitivity to common chemical odours and scents that she used to tolerate, even though she couldn't "prove" it. She had symptoms from her respiratory and central nervous systems, both of which contain TRPV1 receptors. For many years she had worked very close to major traffic and had been subject to long-term exposure to poor air quality. Eventually she became a canary, likely because she always had a poor detoxification system and long-term oxidative stress. Over time this led to sensitized TRPV1 receptors, which explains why she became intolerant to a variety of different, chemically unrelated substances.

Evidence that the brain is involved in MCS is also demonstrated by changes in functional brain scans after chemical exposure. The following summarizes some of the published evidence to support the existence of MCS as a unique, distinct biological entity:

- ☐ The limbic system of the brain contains deposits of chemical pollutants from air pollution
- ☐ Chemicals sensitize the limbic system
- ☐ Chemical pollutant exposure can cause oxidative stress
- ☐ Oxidative stress is common among patients with MCS and SBS, as well as ME/CFS and FM, all of which are frequently co-morbid
- ☐ MCS patients are more likely to have an abnormal genotype for detoxification

☐ MCS patients have inferior detoxification systems compared to the normal population

☐ MCS patients have oxidative stress

☐ Once sensitization to some chemicals occurs, sensitization to other chemicals is more likely

☐ TRPV1 receptors are found in the limbic system of the brain

☐ Sensory neurons contain TRPV1 receptors

☐ TRPV1 receptors are also located in the areas of the body that are dysfunctional in environmentally linked illnesses: the brain, the respiratory system, the gastrointestinal tract, the bladder, and the immune system (mast cells)

☐ Chemicals stimulate TRPV1 receptors

☐ Stimulation of TRPV1 receptors activates neurons

☐ Oxidative stress sensitizes TRPV1 receptors

☐ Chemicals sensitize TRPV1 receptors.

And, most important:

☐ MCS patients have demonstrated TRPV1 receptor sensitization in capsaicin challenge studies.

What all this means is that the sciences of genetics, cell biology, and chemical toxicology, supported by animal models and proper challenge studies in humans, attest to the fact that susceptible people can become sensitized to multiple different chemicals, with resulting illness and disability. This summary of evidence provides very solid proof for the existence of MCS as a distinct biological entity. The weight of evidence is robust. To state that MCS cannot exist because it defies the traditional toxicology paradigm means that it is time for a paradigm shift. The statement "there is no science to support the existence of MCS" now borders on ignorance.

The canaries are real.

CHAPTER 9

CONNECTING THE DOTS

Details create the big picture.

— Sanford I. Weill

My first encounter with environmental medicine was in 1980, with that patient with the thick file who got so much better after Dr. G. treated her for "food allergies." The reason why her chart was so thick was that she had multiple complaints from multiple systems, requiring multiple investigations and multiple consultations with multiple specialists, and costing the provincial medical insurance plan multiple dollars. What I had in her file, but did not recognize at the time, was a pattern of environmentally linked illnesses. What I did not know was that all her symptoms could be traced to shared physiological abnormalities. I will refer to this phenomenon as "the pattern." It is a basket full of common complaints that involve multiple systems.

It was that night in my office in 1985, after examining 200 consecutive charts, that I first noticed the pattern. Since then I have looked for the occurrence of multiple symptoms from multiple systems in every patient. I gathered and developed techniques to sort out all their complaints, the intensity of each, the impact of the complaints on function, and what potentially significant environmental exposures may have occurred. I listened to what the patients were trying to do to reduce symptoms, what worked, and how they coped with their illnesses. I was always intrigued and motivated to try to understand why these phenomena were occurring.

I was seeing new, poorly understood illnesses such as MCS, fibromyalgia, and ME/CFS — vague syndromes with no known or accepted physical cause or verifiable organ changes — that frequently saddled the patients with psychiatric labels. Not only was this not therapeutic, it maligned and discouraged the patients and created obstacles to the emotional support they required from family and friends. It was difficult for them to obtain accommodation at work or financial support from insurers, if the patients were disabled.

Some of the more vocal opponents of environmental medicine pontificated about the lack of evidence for biological illness and accused environmental physicians of quackery. It never occurred to them that they might be wrong, that they could be increasing the patients' psychosocial stress levels and contributing to the severity of their illness.

The Pattern's Components

The brain is the system most commonly affected by environmental illness, leading to complaints of pain, reduced memory and concentration, sleep disturbance, mood changes, and fatigue. Tied for second place in frequency are the respiratory system, with complaints of nasal congestion, postnasal drip, cough and wheeze, and the gastrointestinal system, with symptoms of heartburn, nausea, constipation, diarrhea, gas, abdominal discomfort, and distension. These patients are more likely to have allergies, asthma, eczema, and food, drug, and/or chemical odour intolerances. They are also often sensitive to heat, cold, bright light, noise, and weather changes. They are more likely to have been diagnosed with migraine and/or tension headaches, as well as irritable bowel syndrome. Autoimmune diseases such as psoriasis, lupus, and endometriosis seem to occur more frequently. More than 80 percent are middle-aged women, PMS (premenstrual syndrome) is common, and many of the women are overweight. There is more likely to be a history of a dysfunctional child-hood and a family history of addiction, yet these patients are likely to be very sensitive to or even intolerant of alcohol.

Is this pattern unique? Subjective health complaints or unexplained symptoms are very common, so common that they could be considered almost normal. At least 75 percent of the normal population will have had at least one complaint during the past 30 days from the musculoskel-etal system, gastrointestinal tract, urogenital system, or central nervous system (CNS), with complaints such as fatigue, tiredness, dizziness, and headache. Most people do not seek medical help for these complaints, considering them part of everyday life; the symptoms are mild and very intermittent. Seventy percent of the population perceive their health as very good or excellent. The patients that we see in environmental health clinics, however, have these symptoms more consistently and more se-verely, to the point that their quality of life is significantly affected.

Unexplained symptoms may be common, but the frequency of very substantial complaints — those that occur more frequently and more se-verely — is low. What makes us decide that those symptoms are intoler-able and require help is subjective. There are no obvious cut-off points or apparent thresholds that define the border between what may be simply "normal" complaints and what is intolerable or a significant burden for the patient, both of which indicate possible illness.

One morning my wife woke up to a day scheduled with an import-ant appointment with a client, but she was feeling sick. Determined to attend that meeting, she prepared herself as usual. As we were sitting together at the kitchen table for breakfast, I suggested that she put off the appointment until she was feeling better. She responded by saying that her flu-like symptoms were not so bad and she could still work. She then remarked, "How terrible it must be for your patients to feel like this ev-ery single day!" Where is the disability/severity cut-off point for flu-like symptoms? What if they last for months, or even years?

While most people don't seek medical help for unexplained sub-jective complaints, they are still the most frequent reason for repeated doctor visits and for long-term sickness compensation and permanent inability to work. This has had a very substantial impact on health care budgets and has created significant problems for primary care physicians. It puts a strain on already overburdened family practices. Conflicts may develop when patients consider themselves unable to work because of complaints that are hard to verify objectively, and doctors must rely on the patient's history and subjective evaluation of their ability to work. How do you measure pain and fatigue? How respectful, empathetic, or skeptical is your family doctor?

Understanding Pain

How can anyone understand someone else's pain? How does one describe a sensation to someone who has never had the experience? Words such as *pulling*, *wrenching*, *burning*, *stabbing*, *pinching*, *pressing*, *crushing*, *tight*, and *heavy* are frequently used by patients with chronic musculoskeletal pain, such as in fibromyalgia. If asked to quantify how bad the pain is, most patients use metaphors. The most frequent one I hear in my office is "I feel like I've been run over by a Mack truck." When I respond that I don't know what that feels like and that most people run over by a truck are probably dead, the patients appear to be taken aback.

Since most of my patients are middle-aged women, I ask them if their fibromyalgia pain is equal to the pain of labour. Their answer is that it isn't even close; labour pain is more intense and finite, and there is a baby reward at the end. The pain of fibromyalgia is much milder, but relentless. They are aware of the pain as soon as they wake up and until they fall asleep again, every day. And there is no cure, no reward; medications help only somewhat; and it will never, ever go away. How do you measure that?

Doctors ask patients to rate their pain using a scale of 1 to 10. Most of my patients with fibromyalgia rate their pain as 8 or 9. What is apparent is that one of the major parameters influencing the pain experience is how long they have had it. Recently at a workshop I attended, a frustrated colleague stated that when he described the worst pain as having your limbs removed with a chainsaw without an anesthetic, most of his chronic pain patients reduced their scores to 3 or 4, because their perspective of the pain is affected by its duration. Still, it's all we have, so we use these scales to measure the patients' perspective and to evaluate their response to treatments.

The best way to measure the perception of fatigue or pain is by measuring its impact on daily function and quality of life. Numerous functional assessment questionnaires have been developed and tested for validity and reliability. Unfortunately, most doctors are not familiar with the tools to perform a functional assessment when evaluating disability in chronic illness. Disability should be measured by the impact of the illness on the ability to function. Most physicians have never experienced the continuous symptoms described by their patients. Nevertheless, they are frequently forced to judge the impact of patients' subjective complaints, for which there is no objective evidence. The patients have difficulty describing the pain experience accurately, and the doctors have little training in how to assess the severity of their pain and fatigue.

How patients with multiple subjective complaints are diagnosed depends on the patient's description and the doctor's perception of the illness pattern, plus his or her own belief system regarding etiology, or cause. If the doctor does not accept the existence of MCS, ME/CFS, or fibromyalgia, a psychiatric diagnosis is provided. This is because the symptom pattern frequently overlaps with the diagnostic criteria for disorders such as anxiety, depression, panic disorder, and somatization. If widespread pain or significant fatigue is the main complaint and if the doctor accepts that it is biological, the diagnosis will likely be fibromyalgia or ME/CFS, respectively. It is the physician's paradigm — his or her perception or view of how to explain and understand subjective complaints — that influences the diagnosis, which is then entered in the patients' medical records to follow them for the rest of their lives.

There are no biological markers for any of these disorders, or for psychiatric conditions. The common denominators for all of them are:

- [ ] multiple system complaints
- [ ] oxidative stress
- [ ] central sensitization,
- [ ] multisystem complaints
- [ ] and the pattern.

Teaching in a hospital setting includes discussing each case at the bedside of the patient during rounds. When I was doing my training, if we thought that the patient's symptoms were psychological, we were told to use the word *functional* rather than *psychological*, to be discrete. But for more than a hundred years the word *function* has been used in the medical literature to describe the performance or behaviour of an organ or system; for example, the function of the eye is to see. If you have chronic pain in your leg and there is no clinical evidence of any disease such as arthritis or a broken leg, the pain is considered functional. Unfortunately, we were trained as students to misuse this word. Many physicians interpret *functional* to mean that the cause is psychological, when the fact is all we know is that there is dysfunction.

Multiple chemical sensitivities (MCS), sick building syndrome (SBS), chronic fatigue syndrome (ME/CFS), irritable bowel syndrome (IBS), and fibromyalgia are among those referred to as "functional syndromes" in the medical literature. They are all characterized by frequently overlapping symptoms, suffering, and disabilities, but have no consistent demonstrable tissue abnormality, that is, no objective findings. All we know is that there is dysfunction. There are still many doctors who refer to these conditions as functional in the wrong sense of the word.

All the functional syndromes have variations of the pattern. They share high rates of co-morbidity; in other words, many of the patients have more than one of these diagnoses, but the primary diagnosis given depends on the main complaint. For example, if the main complaint is widespread pain, family doctors may refer the patient to a rheumatologist, and if there are no biological markers, the diagnosis will likely be fibromyalgia. And that patient is very likely to also have chronic fatigue, IBS, sensitivity to chemical odours, and so forth.

Unexplained Functional Syndromes by Specialty

Specialty	Syndrome
Infectious diseases	(Post-viral) Chronic fatigue syndrome
Rheumatology	Fibromyalgia
Otolaryngology	Irritable larynx syndrome
Neurology	Chronic tension headache, chronic migraine
Gastroenterology	Irritable bowel syndrome, dyspepsia
Gynecology	Chronic pelvic pain, vulvodynia
Urology	Interstitial cystitis, painful bladder syndrome, chronic prostatitis
Respirology	Chronic cough
Orthopedics	Chronic low back pain
Cardiology	Atypical chest pain
Psychiatry	Somatoform disorder (hypochondria)
Occupational medicine	Sick building syndrome, multiple chemical sensitivities

Since these entities are frequently co-morbid, there must be a common physiological link. However, many physicians still argue that, in the absence of biological markers, these syndromes are not valid distinct entities — the link is psychiatric. The following analysis comes from the *Annals of Internal Medicine* of the American College of Physicians (1999):

> The suffering of these patients is exacerbated by a self-perpetuating, self-validating cycle in which common, endemic, somatic symptoms are incorrectly attributed to serious abnormality, reinforcing the patient's belief that he or she has a serious disease. Four psychosocial factors propel this cycle of

symptom amplification: the belief that one has a serious disease; the expectation that one's condition is likely to worsen; the "sick role," including the effects of litigation and compensation; and the alarming portrayal of the condition as catastrophic and disabling. The climate surrounding functional somatic syndromes includes sensationalized media coverage, profound suspicion of medical expertise and physicians, the mobilization of parties with a vested self-interest in the status of functional somatic syndromes, litigation, and a clinical approach that overemphasizes the biomedical and ignores psychosocial factors. All of these influences exacerbate and perpetuate the somatic distress of patients with functional somatic syndromes, heighten their fears and pessimistic expectations, prolong their disability, and reinforce their sick role.

I have included the entire excerpt to demonstrate how many arguments can be put forward, without any objective evidence, to strengthen an opinion that is likely wrong. Arguments are made that the patients' perception of their illness is false; that if it is disabling, they are being catastrophic; that the medical component is being overemphasized and the psychosocial factors are being ignored. The opposite position can be — also without any evidence — that the patients' perception is real; that doctors' lack of understanding and supportive care is catastrophic; that the psychosocial factors are being overemphasized and the environmental factors are being ignored. If you are sitting in judgment and there is no evidence, your choice of position will be based on your own paradigm of health. Is it physical or is it mental?

The author of that article is arguing that these unexplained functional syndromes are not separate diagnostic entities. He states that there is one underlying cause.[6] Unfortunately, he concludes that it must be psychiatric. Collapsing them into one psychiatric category enables

6 A.J. Barsky, "Functional somatic syndromes," *Annals of Internal Medecine* 130, no.11 (1999): 910–21.

the author to stay within the old, comfortable paradigm: that if an entity cannot be measured physically, it is mental, and here *functional* means *psychiatric*. Others argue that, even though they have much in common, functional syndromes are not the same but are frequently co-morbid. One thing is clear from the medical literature. Whether we treat these patients symptomatically, using either medications or psychiatric interventions, the therapies are not very successful and many patients are dissatisfied. Since the "it's either physical or mental" approach is not working, we need a new paradigm. That paradigm might be that these are not separate diagnostic entities, that there is one underlying cause but it is not psychological. If so, we need more evidence.

The New Paradigm

Shifting to a new paradigm requires addressing the "it's either physical or mental" argument. The claim that the problem is in the patient's head means that it involves the brain. This actually agrees with the two definitions of *functional* — functional disorders are those arising out of disturbed functioning of the nervous system. But if it is not psychological or psychiatric, if it is not just caused by stress, what is the dysfunction in the nervous system? Also, if these syndromes are really separate entities, what are the common factors that frequently cause people to have more than one of these conditions?

CHAPTER 10

SICK AND TIRED

Health is not valued until sickness comes.

— Thomas Fuller

Are you a healthy, busy, active person? Hopefully you feel valuable, and useful to your family, friends, and co-workers. How would you feel if that was taken away from you because of illness? How unhappy would you feel if you could not participate in the life of your partner or your children the way you used to? Wouldn't you look for the best available medical treatments?

Imagine how frustrating it must be to become chronically ill, only to be told repeatedly that there is nothing physically wrong. Meanwhile, you continue to feel worse. Your job and income are affected yet your symptoms are dismissed as trivial; you are told to "suck it up" and get on with your life.

I see patients every day who have lived this experience. They often express their frustration by saying, "I'm sick and tired of feeling sick and tired." That statement can be found on the tombstone of Fannie Lou Hamer, a black woman who stood up for her rights as an American citizen only to be beaten and abused because of her colour. She remained a civil rights activist until her death. The patients I see who are sick and tired of feeling sick and tired are fighting for their rights as well. While it isn't the same experience, the quote definitely works in this situation. They experience and must fight against prejudicial judgments that make them feel devalued. They are being deprived of accommodation in the workplace and disability benefits. What perpetuates the judgments against them is that their illness is invisible. That they feel sick and tired makes the struggle even harder.

These patients have the pattern, and they frequently meet the criteria for diagnoses of fibromyalgia and chronic fatigue syndrome.

Fibromyalgia

F.J. is a woman in her mid-40s who has experienced widespread chronic pain for three years. The onset was gradual. She described it as a flu-like aching and stiffness in the muscles and joints in her neck, upper and lower back, arms, and legs. Because of the pain she had decreased her time exercising, participating in social activities, and doing hobbies. Her ability to perform household tasks such as cleaning, laundry, and meal preparation was reduced.

F.J. had days of fatigue several times per week, but she felt better if she exercised. Other central nervous system (CNS) complaints included intermittent cognition difficulties such as difficulty finding words, decreased attention span, poor concentration, poor short-term memory, and distractibility. She had been diagnosed with occasional migraines, which occurred once or twice per month. Her sleep pattern was normal but she woke up feeling achy and unrefreshed.

There were no mood changes consistent with anxiety or depression. When she was growing up, her parents often argued, and they divorced when she was nine. She had been sexually abused at age 11 by a neighbour and was in therapy for one year in her early 20s. She worked full-time as a bookkeeper in an accounting firm and was married with three young children.

This patient also had occasional gas and bloating and had been diagnosed with irritable bowel syndrome (IBS). She had allergies to pollens and shellfish and intolerance to alcohol; her occasional hives and asthma required no medication. She also described some chemical odour intolerance: the odours of strongly perfumed products, dry cleaning solvent, deodorizers, fresh paint, and varnish could provoke migraine headaches.

Her environmental exposure history revealed that F.J. worked in a sealed high-rise office building. She had symptoms of itchy eyes and nose, sore throat, hoarse voice, headache, fatigue, and poor concentration when in the workplace, and the symptoms diminished when she left the building. However, there had been no complaints from her colleagues.

She was taking duloxetine, an antidepressant used often for management of chronic pain, which had been somewhat beneficial. Physical examination revealed generalized tenderness. All her blood tests were normal.

F.J. exhibited the typical pattern. Her main complaint was chronic pain but she had multiple system involvement, including the brain, respiratory, gastrointestinal, and immune systems. The brain was the most significant organ system, with pain, cognitive complaints, and sleep disturbance. There was evidence for environmental sensitivity: she had chemical odour intolerance, sick building syndrome, and classical allergies. Her primary diagnosis was fibromyalgia. We measured the impact of her pain on her ability to function, and her score was average for fibromyalgia.

Fibromyalgia is a widespread pain disorder with no biological markers. Since 1990 these have been the most commonly used criteria for the diagnosis of fibromyalgia:

☐ a history of widespread pain that has been present for at least three months (the pain is considered widespread when the following symptoms are present)
☐ pain in both sides of the body

- ☐ pain above and below the waist
- ☐ pain induced by palpation in at least 11 of 18 designated tender point sites.

It has been 20 years since the American College of Rheumatology (ACR) established these diagnostic criteria for fibromyalgia. Because this is a new and evolving area of medicine, the criteria are changing to reflect new information as it becomes available. The ACR is now proposing new diagnostic criteria that remove the absolute requirement for tender points. That criterion had been a factor designed to improve objectivity, but often proved to be a point of contention among physicians. Some doctors did not even look for the tender points, others examined them incorrectly, and some physicians went so far as to refuse to accept the diagnosis as valid if patients were tender in other locations as well. Also, the number of tender points can vary from one appointment to another as severity of the condition fluctuates.

So the rules do need to change. We should remove sole reliance on a mandatory number of tender points and augment them by considering the severity of the widespread pain, fatigue, poor sleep restoration, and cognitive complaints. Spending the time to obtain a more detailed description and measurement of the impact of these complaints seems like a good addition. In fact, it is a distinct improvement because it captures the essence of the condition. It allows doctors to quantify and follow symptom severity. All these criteria and discussions about improvement are being promoted by the ACR, yet the majority of rheumatologists still do not wish to be responsible for the care of patients with fibromyalgia. In fact, more than half of them still believe that fibromyalgia is primarily a psychosomatic illness.

F.J. also met the new criteria for the diagnosis of fibromyalgia. According to the medical literature, this is clearly a central nervous system disorder caused by an abnormality in the mechanism of pain. It involves the limbic system: the peripheral pain receptors have become sensitized and the sensation of pain is maintained by continuous impulses from deep tissues such as muscle and joints, in combination with central sensitization mechanisms.

Central Sensitization

We all have a system for pain, and if all goes well, it is not being activated. When you stub your toe, pain receptors become excited and start transmitting the pain message via the nerves, to the spine and up to the pain centre in the brain, located in the limbic system. Once the message of pain is received, another message is sent back down to the pain receptors in the toe, telling them to turn off. If there is no damage to your toe, the pain goes away. If not, the message will continue cycling until healing takes place. In fibromyalgia the pain receptors are turned on, the message up to the brain is exaggerated, the processing by the limbic system is amplified, and the message to turn off the excited pain receptors is deactivated. This is one wired-up continuous loop. Given that it involves the central nervous system, it is called central sensitization.

Central sensitization is the term used to describe an increased response by the brain to a normal sensory input. It is the exaggerated response to and by a hypersensitive limbic system. This is the part of the brain that receives and responds to all sensory information, helping us read and respond to the environment. When sensitized, the limbic system is likely to overreact to stimulation. We call this tendency hypervigilance.

Central sensitization has been described in several functional disorders besides fibromyalgia. For more than 15 years many researchers have suggested, in reputable journals such as the *Annals of the New York Academy of Sciences*, that central sensitization is the physiological explanation for MCS. The theory had been considered unproven until recently. Studies now provide strong objective evidence for the occurrence of central sensitization in MCS.

It is no surprise that F.J. also had MCS. Central sensitization occurs in fibromyalgia, MCS, migraine, and IBS. It is one of the mechanisms responsible for manifestation of the pattern, and it explains the pattern seen in F.J.'s medical history.

Central sensitization turns on an exaggerated sensory pathway for pain, with an exaggerated response to any mild stimuli. Some patients with fibromyalgia find that even tight clothing hurts. This is because the perception of pain is so amplified that even stimuli not normally perceived as painful initiate a sensation of pain. A heightened response to painful stimulation is also present. It is like turning up a volume control setting too high.

The pain pathway is connected by the limbic system to the cortex, producing our conscious awareness of painful sensations. We are more irritable when we have pain. Emotions stimulate this pain pathway by their impact on an already hypervigilant limbic system. Stress influences pain, and vice versa.

Limbic Connection to Pain Disorders

The limbic system in the brain processes and responds to all the information we can receive from the environment. Sensations such as touch and pain are managed by the limbic system, which also regulates sleep according to daylight. Therefore people with chronic pain disorders, who have an overstimulated and dysfunctional limbic system, will frequently have sleep disturbance and fatigue, just like F.J. These factors are now part of the new criteria for the diagnosis of fibromyalgia. Limbic system dysfunction is why F.J. has chemical sensitivities: her limbic system has become sensitized to chemicals in the environment.

Patients with fibromyalgia frequently have alterations in mood because the limbic system is intricately involved in the dynamics of mood expression. They are more likely to have had, or presently to have, major depression and panic disorder. Having a history of depression is a risk factor for fibromyalgia.

F.J. underwent successful psychotherapy in her early 20s because of child abuse. Could that history of abuse have played a role in her later development of fibromyalgia? For 15 years, abuse in childhood — emotional, physical, and sexual — has been researched as a potential cause of fibromyalgia. This hypothesis assumes that there is a link in the brain between abuse and the mechanisms of pain. However, the studies have come to different conclusions. The quality of the studies was generally poor, and combining the results demonstrates only modest associations between chronic pain and having been abused or neglected in childhood. Nevertheless there is a possibility that a history of sexual abuse can contribute to the development of fibromyalgia. This is used unfairly to lend support to the argument that unexplained chronic pain is caused by psychiatric illness. Contribution and cause are not the same.

There is an abundance of literature describing the psychological impact of child abuse. When patients complain of physical pain without abnormal objective tests to substantiate it, doctors consider the possibility of psychiatric illness. When doctors use a narrow, reductionist[7] paradigm and lack a sufficient understanding of the function of the limbic system, they are much more likely to apply a psychiatric label and to dismiss other potential functional, biological contributors and causes.

Child abuse does not cause just emotional dysfunction. It causes both physical and functional abnormalities in the structures of the developing brain, particularly in the limbic system. What constitutes child abuse? Sexual or physical abuse is clear, but there is a lack of consensus regarding the definition of emotional abuse. According to the World Health Organization, up to 85 percent of parents yell at their children, so where do we draw the line between normal and abnormal parenting?

When patients come to my office for the first time, they fill out a very lengthy questionnaire. One section deals with stress. I ask if there is a history of emotional, physical, or sexual abuse. I also ask them to de-

7 An attempt to understand the interactions of complex phenomena by reducing them down to one simple explanation. See chapter 14 for an in-depth examination of reductionist thinking.

scribe their childhoods, whether they were normal, happy, unhappy, or stressful. Sometimes they deny any abuse yet check off "unhappy" and/ or "stressful." This gives me an opportunity to explore childhood issues. Sometimes the issue was bullying, but I am much more likely to hear "I never got along with my mother because she was so critical [or controlling]," or "My father was an alcoholic," or "My parents fought a lot."

Children do not have to be beaten or raped for stress to affect them. Long-standing childhood stress can have an impact on the developing brain similar to that of abuse, causing a permanent hypervigilant condition in the limbic system. This explains why adult patients with a chronic pain disorder exhibit higher levels of pain when they also have a history of child abuse.

From a developmental, evolutionary, and survival point of view, these biological changes in the brain are adaptive responses to an early environment characterized by threat. An abused child adapts biologically to survive in response to the challenges posed by his or her surroundings. Early stress programs the hard wiring of the brain to meet the demands of a hostile environment. These patients develop patterns of hypervigilance, both emotionally and biologically. Learned hypervigilance is an adaptive response to living in an unpredictable home environment, and the changes persist. The child learns to watch out and be careful both emotionally and structurally. Psychotherapy can attenuate and reduce behavioural and emotional issues that develop as a consequence of child abuse. It can improve function of the neurons.

Can psychotherapy remove developmental structural abnormalities in the brain? The answer is that we don't know yet. But consider the following. Evidence is emerging for child abuse having long-term effects on physical health over a lifetime. Warm, nurturing families tend to promote resistance to stress and to diminish vulnerability to stress-induced illness. But by midlife, individuals who rate their relationship with parents as cold and detached have a fourfold greater risk of chronic illness, including heart disease and diabetes.

This is what the medical literature tells us: we know there is an association of child abuse with being overweight or obese as an adult, which we can easily attribute to emotionally driven poor diet choices and overeating. But perhaps this explanation is incomplete. Other hormone factors may be involved, because child abuse puts people at risk to develop diabetes, independent of weight gain. Adult victims of child abuse are more likely to develop chronic lung disease, and smoking explains only part of that increase. They are more likely to develop asthma. They are also at risk to develop cardiovascular disease and autoimmune disorders and to experience premature mortality.

You don't have to be overweight to have a heart attack, but it increases the odds, as does being significantly stressed in childhood. Similarly, you don't have to have been abused in childhood to develop fibromyalgia, but it can be a contributing factor. There is also some evidence that child abuse can be a predisposing factor in chronic fatigue syndrome (ME/CFS).

Clearly, using psychotherapy and psychotherapeutic medications alone is not an appropriate primary treatment for patients with cardiovascular disease, asthma, diabetes, or autoimmune disorder who have a childhood history of abuse. It doesn't work for fibromyalgia, ME/CFS, and MCS either.

Chronic Fatigue Syndrome

O.C. is a 47-year-old woman who was referred to me because of fatigue for the previous eight years. For her, the fatigue started with a viral infection from which she never fully recovered. After a few months she had recovered sufficiently to be able to return to work. In order to do so, she had to reduce her social activities and had to hire someone to help her with household chores. Her husband took over meal preparation for the whole family. She no longer exercised to the extent that she had prior to the viral infection because it would aggravate the fatigue, even into the next day. She limited her exercise to walking the dog in the evenings with her husband, although sometimes she was too tired to do even that.

She always felt as if she had the flu, feeling achy and irritable. She had used occasional sick days to rest, but her fatigue gradually became worse and her muscle pain increased. A rheumatologist diagnosed her with fibromyalgia. O.C. tried several medications and eventually settled on duloxetine, the antidepressant commonly used for pain disorders. This reduced but did not stop her pain.

O.C. described her marriage as happy; her husband was caring and supportive. There were no financial worries and her children were busy academically and socially. She liked her job as a department manager and her boss was supportive in trying to accommodate her. She described her childhood as happy and normal.

She associated the worsening of her fatigue and pain with the development of another issue. There were ongoing renovations in the office tower where she worked, which had a shopping mall on the first floor. Shortly after arriving there she would develop symptoms of itchy eyes, nasal congestion, sore throat, hoarse voice, cough, poor concentration, and a mentally dull feeling. Her face felt hot and she looked flushed. Her fatigue and muscle aches would increase and she would develop a dull headache. These symptoms would start slowly, within a few minutes of arriving at work, and could be relieved by going outside, depending on the severity and duration of exposure. Her recovery time was relatively short when she first began to have these reactions at work, but gradually it became longer and longer. She began to notice aggravation of these symptoms by exposure to perfumed products worn by some of her colleagues, as well as the odours of fresh paint, deodorizers, detergents, soaps, and fabric softeners.

O.C. had a long-standing history of allergies to pollens and was taking allergy shots. She was also allergic to codeine. She had gastrointestinal complaints and her gastroenterologist had diagnosed her with irritable bowel syndrome (IBS).

O.C. had the pattern. She had the central nervous system complaints of fatigue, pain, and poor cognition, respiratory symptoms, and gastrointestinal complaints. But what was happening to her biologically? She was tired and achy when she went back to work and likely already had central sensitization. This made her prone to becoming sensitized to environmental factors, which is exactly what happened because of the repeated exposure to indoor pollutants from the renovations at work: now she had sick building syndrome. The repeated chemical exposures increased the hits to her limbic system. As a result, she developed more pain and fatigue and became sensitized to more chemicals, such as the scented products of her co-workers. She had become a canary.

O.C. came to see me because she felt she could no longer work. Her fatigue would be worse by the end of the day and she could no longer recover by the next day. She spent most of the weekends just resting, and her quality of life had clearly deteriorated. However, her insurance carrier denied her disability because of "lack of clinical evidence that the symptoms limited her ability to perform the essentials of her job."

Physical examination and laboratory tests found no abnormalities. Her diagnoses were chronic fatigue syndrome, fibromyalgia, sick building syndrome, and multiple chemical sensitivities. We measured the impact of the fatigue and pain on function by using standardized questionnaires. The results were significantly abnormal, which validated her disability for work.

I prepared a report for her insurance company and provided the results of the functional assessment, as well as the following information, supported by citations from the medical literature. The level of disability and her inability to perform the essentials of her job were worsened because three different conditions were involved: ME/CFS, fibromyalgia, and MCS. They created synergistic negative effects on the same area of the brain — the limbic system. Studies show that the scores measuring disability are usually worse if multiple diseases are present. Patients with ME/CFS report significant and disabling cognitive difficulties such as impaired concentration, made worse by chemical triggers, and patients with ME/CFS are more likely to develop MCS. The majority of patients with ME/CFS experience chronic widespread pain. People with ME/CFS, fibromyalgia, or MCS endure significant disability in terms of physical, occupational, and social functioning, and those with more than one of these diagnoses report greater severity of physical and mental fatigue. Most patients with ME/CFS are unemployable. Ultimately the insurance carrier reversed its decision and granted O.C. her disability benefits.

The diagnosis of ME/CFS is made primarily by exclusion. There are no definitive laboratory tests or physical findings, but what distinguishes it from other causes of chronic fatigue is that it is made worse by exertion and not substantially relieved by rest, and post-exertion recovery time is prolonged. Sometimes it can take days or weeks to recover, instead of minutes or hours. The fatigue in ME/CFS is both physical and cognitive, and it rarely goes away. This is the reason why so many of these patients are disabled.

The various definitions of ME/CFS often contain other symptoms and patterns, including chronic pain (such as recurrent headaches and widespread pain), disturbed or less than refreshing sleep, cognitive complaints, gastrointestinal complaints, and sensitivities to foods, medications, odours, and/or chemicals. Note the same recurrent pattern: multiple system complaints involving the brain. There is increasing evidence for the role of central sensitization. As well, the immune system appears to be playing a role in the dysfunction of ME/CFS. And there is even more robust evidence for oxidative stress.

Oxidative stress causes changes in muscle cell function, which is not surprising, since oxidative stress occurs easily in muscles. Their antioxidant defence mechanisms are generally poor. Exercise studies on ME/CFS patients show reduced muscle excitability and impaired recovery, and simultaneous increases in oxidative stress. ME/CFS patients produce more metabolic by-products from exercise compared to normal individuals, and they have reduced mitochondrial function.

The explanation for the condition has to do with oxidative stress and subsequent reduction in mitochondrial function. The evidence for oxidative stress in ME/CFS is robust. The reason that it has become more prevalent in the past 30 years is clearly environmental.

ME/CFS and Exercise

Several studies of ME/CFS have used cardiopulmonary exercise testing. In this test, the patient exercises to the maximum, usually on a treadmill or stationary bicycle, while heart and lung functions are monitored. The test ends when the individual can no longer continue to exercise or when the physician has gathered enough information. It is most often used to diagnose or rule out coronary artery disease.

Patients with ME/CFS usually score the same as normal sedentary people of the same age. However, repeating the exercise test on the following day shows a difference. Healthy people demonstrate the same exercise capacity the next day, but patients with ME/CFS have a reduced capacity because their recovery from exertion is prolonged. This provides objective evidence of a biological abnormality in energy production.

Exercise studies on ME/CFS patients demonstrate impaired recovery and simultaneous increases in oxidative stress. They also show that they have reduced mitochondrial function and produce more metabolic by-products from exercise when compared to normal individuals. This is why they have fatigue with prolonged recovery. Pushing these patients to exercise beyond their limits makes them worse.

ME/CFS and Depression

ME/CFS patients have an increased prevalence of current and lifetime mood disorders, primarily major depression. Some doctors use this fact to insist that ME/CFS is primarily a psychiatric illness. There is reason for the confusion; numerous studies demonstrate that patients with depression also have significantly elevated markers of oxidative damage, and the severity of depression correlates with the magnitude of the oxidative stress disturbance.

Could depression and ME/CFS be the same entity? They each have the diagnostic criteria of physical and mental fatigue and co-morbid disorders of sleep disturbance, pain, gastrointestinal disturbances, and immunologic abnormalities. They both demonstrate oxidative stress.

We know that patients with ME/CFS have poorer muscle performance and an abnormal brain response as measured by electroencephalogram (EEG), compared to healthy controls. They also have decreased cognition, although not as badly as those who are depressed. Sleep patterns differ. Brain scans can demonstrate abnormalities in chronic fatigue syndrome patients that differ from depression. There are numerous subjective differences between ME/CFS and depression, as illustrated in the following table.

	ME/CFS	Depression
Exercise	Exacerbates fatigue	Feeling better after exercise
Sleep	Less than refreshing or excessive	Insomnia or excessive
Fatigue-associated symptoms	Frustration	Apathy
Symptom interpretation	Less likely in terms of negative emotions	More likely in terms of negative emotions
Illness attribution	External or somatic experiences	Psychological factors (maybe)
Coping	More likely by limiting activities	More likely by increasing activities

What all these findings demonstrate is that ME/CFS is a unique entity, different from depression. While there are no diagnostic markers for ME/CFS, there are no diagnostic markers for depression either. A physician must be both knowledgeable and experienced to be able to differentiate between them in order to make the correct diagnosis.

A few years ago I gave a workshop to family physicians on how to assess function in patients with ME/CFS and fibromyalgia. Among those attending was a medical advisor for the Canada Pension Plan (CPP) disability benefits program. To my surprise he volunteered that ME/CFS was the result of women having joined the workforce, but that they were too ambitious and competitive and thus eventually burned out. When I responded that there was no good literature to support that opinion, he disagreed, citing one article. His position was sexist and, given that more than half the attending doctors were female, an animated dialogue ensued, making my workshop a dynamic success.

ME/CFS and burnout are not the same. Burnout is a persistent negative work-related state of mind. Symptoms include emotional exhaustion, feelings of distress, reduced effectiveness, decreased motivation, and dysfunctional, negative attitudes and behaviours at work. These symptoms are mostly psychological, and workers who are burned out are most likely to attribute their complaints to problems at work, blaming their job for their condition. Fatigue is a predominant complaint. Burnout patients also have EEG abnormalities that differ from ME/CFS, and they do not have the same pattern of fatigue.

After the workshop I approached the physician from the CPP. I told him that if my patients applied for disability I advised them to expect rejection by the CPP, even after they appealed. I encourage them to appeal again, to the Pensions Appeal Board, because then they will likely be accepted. My colleagues and I have found that denial or delay of the disability pension is very stressful for patients who have no income and cannot ever work again, and that the present system makes the patients physically worse. I asked the physician to explain why this occurred almost routinely. He smiled and responded that, in the end, it was judges, not doctors, who made the final decision. A few months later we approached the CPP physicians via the College of Family Physicians and suggested bringing together the college and CPP physicians in a workshop to try to resolve this dilemma. They refused, claiming that they had their own medical resources for information on ME/CFS. Resistance in the medical profession takes many forms.

This experience shows the potential for harm when those in a position of power and responsibility are biased and misinformed. When they are stuck in a box and incapable of engaging in dialogue with their own peers, they cannot have the public's best interests in mind. It also raises another salient point. It is not sufficient to simply identify a pattern of symptoms and dysfunction; a diagnosis must be established to predict the prognosis. Only patients who will likely never recover qualify for CPP disability. Burnout or depression patients have a better prognosis for recovery; they usually recover sufficiently, whereas most ME/CFS patients do not.

CHAPTER 11

MORE DOTS TO CONNECT

Vision is the art of seeing what is invisible to others.

— Jonathan Swift

D.M. is a high-functioning mother and wife and runs her own business. She had frequent headaches, shoulder pain, and heartburn. When she came to see me because of increasing chemical sensitivities, she had been taking over-the-counter (OTC) pain medications and antacids for more than 20 years. "I just pop a pill and get on with it."

Most people with the pattern consider themselves healthy. You do not have to be disabled with fibromyalgia or ME/CFS when you have it. There is a spectrum of complaints, and mild pain or fatigue can still be part of the pattern. Maybe you don't see yourself as having a chronic pain issue because you can control it with analgesics. This happens frequently. Pain relievers as a group have the highest sales among OTC drugs. In the United States, 9 to 13 billion tablets of acetaminophen are used annually, amounting to 50 to 70 tablets per person per year. Pain seems to be a problem even in people who consider themselves healthy.

When patients have pain and all the tests come back negative, doctors still need to label the condition. Using the description of the pain provided by the patient, the doctor provides an appropriate diagnosis. The common ones are described in this chapter. As you read through these chronic pain conditions, you might recognize yourself, a family member, or a friend. Even if you are reassured about the benign nature of the episodes of pain, you should not accept this situation blindly without considering the dynamics behind it. Is there evidence for the pattern? Are you developing a hypervigilant limbic system, central sensitization, and oxidative stress? Are you becoming the next canary?

Chronic Migraine Headaches

Migraine is usually a debilitating headache. The pain can be so severe that it can disrupt work, time with family, and social life. People take a pill for the headache when required, or more regularly to prevent recurrent migraines. The cost to the medical system is low; however, the cost to society of absence from work and reduced productivity is considerable.

The diagnosis of migraine is based on clinical history, because there are no biological markers or specific clinical tests. Most common are episodic migraines, which are characterized by headaches that last 4 to 72 hours. Patients typically describe the pain as unilateral (on one side), pulsating, moderate or severe, aggravated by routine physical activity, and associated with nausea and/or bright light and noise.

Chronic migraines are more debilitating. Considered chronic if they occur at least 15 days per month, they are different from the occasional episodic migraines because when they develop, there are measurable changes in the limbic system, with robust evidence for central sensitization. The pain system is turned on in these patients. Currently migraine is considered a continuum or spectrum disorder, because people with episodic migraines are more likely to develop chronic migraine headaches and central sensitization.

Chronic Tension Headache

Tension headache is the most common headache type worldwide, and most people do not seek medical attention unless it becomes frequent and debilitating. It is usually bilateral and feels like a pressure or tightening in the head, sometimes accompanied by nausea. Just like chronic migraines, tension headaches are labelled as chronic when they occur 15 or more days per month for at least six months. Tension headaches can be caused by muscle contraction in the head and neck, but chronic tension headaches are due to a turned-on pain system. Studies now confirm the association of these chronic headaches with central sensitization.

Chronic Low Back Pain

The lifetime incidence of low back pain is between 50 and 80 percent of the population, and it often follows a prolonged course of recurring episodes and remissions. It is a musculoskeletal disorder that is often caused by muscle overuse or strain sustained over a period of time. It is thought to be due to mechanical causes. The definition of chronic low back pain is established by persistence of the pain beyond three or six months, depending on which studies you read. When it becomes chronic, central sensitization is playing a role.

Rheumatic (Immune) Diseases

Rheumatic diseases are inflammatory conditions that involve muscles and joints, such as rheumatoid arthritis, endometriosis, and lupus. Because widespread pain is generated by the inflammation, the pain system is constantly being stimulated. Therefore we see central sensitization occurring more frequently in rheumatic diseases.

Osteoarthritis

Osteoarthritis is a common progressive deterioration of joints associated with aging, obesity, and family history. Pain is the most common symptom, but it does not correspond well with the X-ray findings, which usually don't look as bad as the patient feels. Several studies of osteoarthritis have demonstrated the presence of hyperalgesia (abnormal pain sensitivity) with central sensitization. My mother, who was healthy for 95 years, had significant osteoarthritis in her hands. She needed to use both hands to hold a glass of water because she could not grip it with her fingers. She had minimal pain and took no medication — she did not have central sensitization.

Chronic Pelvic Pain

Chronic pelvic pain affects nine million women in the United States. Doctors often tell these women that nothing can be done and that the cause is unknown. Approximately 40 percent of gynecological laparoscopies are performed to assess chronic pelvic pain, but they find no pathology in 35 percent of them. Several common, difficult-to-treat conditions — such as vulvodynia, painful menstruation, interstitial cystitis/painful bladder syndrome, and, in men, chronic prostatitis — fall under the umbrella of chronic pelvic pain.

Vulvodynia is a chronic type of pain that affects the female external genital area (vulva) and has no identifiable cause or visible pathology. I once had a patient whose husband drove her 1,500 kilometres to see me because she had vulvodynia. It was so painful for her to sit for long periods that she lay on the back seat of the car with her feet out the window, wearing a skirt in order to get relief from the cool air.

Although this was an extreme case, this condition affects approximately 16 percent of women. The most common description is burning pain, but others have described it as knifelike or like acid being poured on the skin. Sex is painful, and the pain can be provoked by anything that exerts pressure on the area, such as tampon insertion, speculum examination by a physician, riding a bike, or even sitting for a long period of time. Vulvodynia is a complex regional pain syndrome caused by central sensitization.

Primary dysmenorrhea (painful menstruation) is menstrual pain without any pelvic abnormality, and it is the most common gynecological disorder in women of child-bearing age, especially in adolescence. These women display evidence of central sensitization that is maintained throughout the entire menstrual cycle, even in the absence of pain.

Chronic prostatitis is a pelvic pain in men. Whether or not the pain is generated by the prostate is not clear. The pain can be felt in the testicles, penis, lower abdomen, or perineum (the area between the scrotum and the anus in men, or the vagina and the anus in women). Urination or ejaculation may intensify the pain. The cause is unknown and attempts to find prostate pathology have failed. Nonetheless, there are many men with this condition whose lives have been dramatically altered because of reduced physical activity, social life, and sexual activity. The studies show that these men demonstrate central sensitization.

Interstitial cystitis/painful bladder syndrome is a group of symptoms that include decreased bladder capacity; an urgent need to urinate frequently, day and night; feelings of pressure, pain, and tenderness around the bladder, pelvis, and perineum; painful sexual intercourse; and discomfort in the penis or scrotum. This disorder is another confirmation of central sensitization. I see it frequently in my practice and consider it part of the pattern.

Irritable Bowel Syndrome and Reflux

Irritable bowel syndrome (IBS) is a very common gastrointestinal (GI) motility disorder, occurring in up to 23 percent of the population. It is most commonly diagnosed when cramping, abdominal pain, bloating, constipation, and/or diarrhea occur frequently in the absence of any abnormal tests. Two-thirds of these patients report food intolerances, although for many reasons, food challenge studies have varied widely in their support.

The distress caused by the symptoms of IBS ranges from mildly abnormal stool production to significant pain and impact on function. It ranges from the physical discomfort of abdominal bloating and flatulence to severe urgency to defecate. This urgency can result in frustration during simple everyday tasks such as standing in line at the bank. For some people IBS can be so disabling that they may be unable to work, attend social events, or even travel short distances because of pain or the urgency to defecate. I once had a patient who was on disability for severe IBS because his job was to lead canoe trips. Patients with IBS must often plan the events of their day according to the availability of toilets. Paradoxically, IBS also includes the other end of the spectrum: constipation.

Many patients feel that IBS is a "garbage-can diagnosis" because the doctor can't find anything wrong. This is because X-rays, scans, and scopes do not show the movements of the intestine. IBS is a disorder of bowel wall movements. If food travels through the gastrointestinal system too quickly, the water used to help digest it is not reabsorbed enough, and we pass a watery, poorly formed stool, which we call diarrhea. If it goes through too slowly, we are constipated. We can detect disorders in gut motility in research labs, using swallowed radio-opaque markers and special cameras to follow them.

As we digest food, the gastrointestinal system moves it along with a rhythmical series of contractions, normally in one direction. This is called peristalsis. It occurs because the mass of food distends the gut, stretching its walls, and neurological sensors assess the stretching. When the nervous system senses enough stretching, a reflex response initiates contraction. The sensitivity of those sensors (the neurological response) and the subsequent reflex contractions dictate whether the movements of the intestinal wall are normal, overreacting (causing diarrhea), or under-reacting (causing constipation).

IBS is also more common in patients with chronic fatigue syndrome and chronic pain disorders such as fibromyalgia and chronic pelvic pain. Many IBS patients also have motility problems in the upper digestive system, causing stomach acid to flow back into the esophagus, with heartburn as the result. This is called gastroesophageal reflux disease (GERD), and it often coexists with IBS because they share the same abnormal mechanism of dysmotility.

In the past two decades there has been a surge of research in the area of motility, brain imaging, and neurotransmitters. This research has helped define the brain–gut axis, the bidirectional connection between the brain and the GI tract — systems communicating with systems. The limbic system is abnormal in IBS and there is evidence for central sensitization.

We are familiar with the "butterflies in the stomach" metaphor: that sensation felt in anticipation of a stressful event. The medical literature also connects anxiety and depression with IBS. Psychosocial factors can play a vital role at any and all stages in the patient's history and can actually predispose people to IBS and GERD. They influence the brain's impact on the sensory and motor dysfunction of the GI tract. However, the brain–gut axis works both ways, since it is bidirectional.

The connection of the brain with the GI tract is extensive and includes the limbic system, which reads the environment of the intestine from the messages received via the sensors on the nerve endings. Hypersensitive responses to the sensors in the bowel and abnormal pain processing cause the major clinical features of IBS: abnormal bowel movements and abdominal cramps and pain. Remember the TRPV1 receptors we were talking about with MCS? They exist in the bowel as well. Activation of abnormal TRPV1 receptors, as well as central sensitization, occurs in irritable bowel syndrome. This helps to explain why IBS and GERD are also more common in patients with multiple chemical sensitivities and why my patient D.M. developed MCS too.

IBS and the Immune System

Inflammatory bowel diseases such as Crohn's disease and ulcerative colitis occur because the immune system attacks the bowel. We refer to these types of diseases as autoimmune because the immune system is attacking one's own body, in this case the lining of the bowel. The inflammation in the bowel lining is visible to the gastroenterologist when he performs a colonoscopy. Redness, swelling, and pathological changes can be seen. Under a microscope one can even see many immune system cells crowded into the damaged tissues. Normally, healthy tissues have a few immune system cells lurking about, screening the environment and looking for bad guys — foreign molecules that they don't recognize. When danger is detected, these few immune cells call in reinforcements by releasing chemical messengers called cytokines. Other immune cells are then attracted to the area, contributing to the inflammatory response.

This inflammation is not visible in IBS, visually or under the microscope, and until recently it was thought not to be present. However, the IBS literature now provides strong evidence for immune system involvement. We can now measure elevated levels of cytokines in the wall of the intestine in IBS, especially when the patient is reacting to some food intolerance.

For many years my patient R.S. had symptoms of itchy eyes, rhinitis, and asthma from April to July because of grass and tree pollen allergies. He also had severe IBS symptoms during that same pollen season, until he was desensitized to the pollens by allergy shots. Patients with allergies are more likely to have IBS. IBS patients who also have allergies have more severe IBS symptoms, and even higher levels of cytokines. The link is central sensitization in the limbic system, which causes hypervigilant environmental surveillance. This leads to excessive responses to environmental factors by the sensors in the intestinal wall, the pain receptors, and the cells of the immune system.

IBS is more than a garbage-can diagnosis for doctors when they can't find anything wrong clinically. It is a complex condition. On an organ level, IBS involves interactions of the gastrointestinal, nervous, and immune systems. On a cellular level, there is evidence for oxidative stress, and on a molecular level, there are more cytokines — those pro-inflammatory chemical mediators. And IBS is frequently co-morbid with other chronic conditions. Many studies of patients with ME/CFS and fibromyalgia indicate that they frequently have IBS. More than two-thirds of patients diagnosed with IBS in GI clinics have accompanying chronic fatigue and widespread pain.

Once again we see that same pattern of multiple system complaints and multi-morbidity. Patients who exhibit the pattern have chronically higher levels of cytokines and oxidative stress, and most patients who have IBS also have the symptoms of the pattern.

Immune System Messaging

When the immune system is challenged by a foreign invader (bacteria or virus) or an injury, it calls for help from other immune cells. Cytokines are released to stimulate the immune system's response of coming to the rescue. Cytokines also communicate with the limbic system to let it know what is going on. A variety of chemical, hormonal, and behavioural changes occur in response. This signalling is part of a generalized, comprehensive mechanism that all animals have that mobilizes the whole body to respond to any perceived physical and/or psychological stress. The immune system influences the brain, in particular the limbic system, and a stress response by the brain also mobilizes the immune system. They work together and support each other as a team.

One of my first epiphanies was in the 1980s, with the toy store cashier who was actually an experimental psychologist. He enlightened me about the concepts of psychoneuroimmunology, a concept that conventional allergists were resisting. Today researchers accept that activation of immune cells results in changes in brain function. That is what causes us to feel sickness.

Sickness Behaviour

Everyone has experienced an episode of viral or bacterial infection, with its accompanying feelings of sickness such as malaise, lethargy, fatigue, muscle and joint aches, and reduced appetite. We think of these symptoms as trivial components of the process affecting sick individuals, but the emotional and behavioural components of sickness are actually a highly organized purposeful way of fighting infection. All animals behave this way when they are sick; it is not by choice and it is not psychological.

Sickness behaviour is the behavioural component of illness. Cytokines, produced by activated immune system cells, trigger it. Sick individuals have little motivation to eat, are listless, complain of fatigue and malaise, lose interest in social activities, and have significant changes in sleep patterns. They display an inability to experience pleasure, have exaggerated responses to pain, and fail to concentrate. These nearly universal behavioural changes are designed to promote recovery. We don't behave that way on purpose.

Sickness behaviour is physiological, like other motivational states such as fear, hunger, and thirst. It is a behaviour motivated by the biological need to take care of ourselves, a basic instinct for survival. It is normal to withdraw from the environment and to seek rest and care for the body in response to infection. It is as normal as shifting to a state of increased arousal and readiness for action when confronted with a potential threat, and as normal as seeking water or food when we are thirsty or hungry. This is an adaptive response to infection or trauma. Cytokine release is the immune system's way of telling the brain to minimize the activity of all the other organs, to stay quiet, to use a minimum amount of energy, allowing the immune system to use whatever energy resources are required to fight the invading organisms.

Sickness behaviour overlaps with the symptoms of depression, including depressed mood, reduced social interaction, and sleep disturbance. Cytokines have an impact on limbic system function and can influence emotions. Clinical studies have shown increased levels of cytokines in the blood of depressed patients. This is probably why patients who suffer from chronic inflammatory conditions are more likely to be depressed. They aren't just feeling sorry for themselves; cytokines can themselves provoke or exacerbate mood disorders. Several experiments were performed on healthy volunteers to whom cytokines were administered intravenously. Doing so caused flu-like symptoms, followed by depression. Cytokines are elevated in depressed patients, and they can also predict the onset of a depressive episode.

The release of cytokines can even be triggered by air pollution. This emphasizes the environmental connection to illness behaviours and depressive symptoms, a connection that is often missed, ignored, or denied. Air pollution can increase the emotional symptoms of depression, especially in the elderly. Several studies have found a connection between air pollution and a rise in emergency department visits because of depression and suicide attempts.

Connect the Dots and Get the Picture

The environment can influence or cause illness. But this is obvious only to people who can feel the reactions induced by chemical exposures — the canaries. Chemical exposures increase the burden on our detoxification systems, causing or exacerbating oxidative stress. This exposure can adversely affect many illnesses in which oxidative stress is occurring. Chemical exposures and oxidative stress activate TRPV1 receptors, which are found on the membranes of cells of the immune, respiratory, gastrointestinal, and central nervous systems — the systems involved in the pattern.

The environment can affect our mood and behaviour biologically, even making us suicidal. It can contribute to cardiovascular disease, respiratory illness, allergies and autoimmune diseases, chronic pain, and gastrointestinal dysfunction. Each of the systems involved interacts with the others. They do so via the limbic system, cytokines, and TRPV1 receptors.

These are the common denominators that explain the functional disorders, and the environment influences them.

If you're a canary you can feel it. If you aren't, you can't.

PART IV

THE ENVIRONMENTAL LINK WITH CHRONIC ILLNESS

NAME_____ AGE_____

ADDRESS_____ DATE_____

☐ LABEL

REFILL 0 1 2 3 4 5   _____

                                      (SIGNATURE)

CHAPTER 12

THE BODY'S NATURAL DEFENCE SYSTEM

The problem in defence is how far you can go without destroying from within what you are trying to defend from without.

— Dwight D. Eisenhower

Every organism needs a defence system for protection, and ours is the immune system. It is like a national security system, protecting us from invasion by parasites, bacteria, and viruses and responding to any perceived attack, such as a laceration or trauma, with an inflammatory response. It has memory and an excellent filing system, keeping track of and recording information on whatever it encounters, for future reference. It is capable of recognizing what is normal in the environment, such as our own tissues and organs, the foods that enter our bodies through digestion, and the usual pollens and spores that we inhale.

The immune system is also present to protect us from invading microbes. Microbes are parasites, bacteria, and viruses. They exist everywhere, and on every surface. Not all of them have the potential to cause illness but some have the potential to invade the body, or overcome the body's defences, if given the opportunity. Some can cause damage by releasing toxins and harmful enzymes.

The immune system can be divided in two: the more primitive innate immune system, which is built-in, and the acquired system, which is more evolutionarily advanced. The acquired system develops and matures through our experiences as we encounter various microbes. It has a fantastic memory and learns to recognize specific foreign invaders that it has met and dealt with previously, and therefore it can respond much more quickly.

A healthy immune system is programmed to recognize the cells belonging to the body it protects and to leave them alone. It does so by recognizing markers on the cell membranes and being able to distinguish between itself and foreign cells. When immune system defenders encounter cells with markers recognized as foreign, it stimulates a response.

Microbes and Our Environment

Microbes are everywhere and are constantly being screened by the immune system. They are part of our personal environment. We generally consider ourselves to be clean, but complex mixtures of microbes are constant residents in all our orifices, on our skin and respiratory tract lining, and in the lower intestine. The vast collection of microbes that live on and inside us is called the microbiota, and collectively its gene pool is known as the microbiome.

Scientists are able to study microbial communities by examining genetic material. For years the only way they were able to examine the microbiota was by culturing a swab in a lab and examining the material under a microscope. Through advancement in medical technology, they now have procedures that allow them to look at the microbial community inside the human body, and they have found a much greater diversity in the microbial world than they previously thought existed.

The intestine has the largest and densest collection of organisms in the human microbiome; in fact, the intestinal microbiome is the most biologically dense niche known. Investigators have estimated that the gastrointestinal tract in an adult human contains approximately 500 to 1,000 distinct bacterial species. Altogether, there are 100 trillion organisms in the intestine, most of which are bacteria, which is astounding, considering that the entire human body is made up of only three trillion cells. The genetic material from these bacteria represents 100 times more genes than the entire human genome.

According to evolutionary theory, species with the greatest ability to survive will increase in abundance, regardless of the consequences on other species. Organisms can also incidentally contribute to the success and survival of other species. When this happens in a reciprocal manner, it is referred to as mutualistic. Our relationship with our own microbiota is mutualist. It is part of our environment, and when we tamper with the balance, there can be repercussions and unintended consequences. For example, taking antibiotics can alter the balance of the microbiota and cause symptoms of IBS.

We have a symbiotic mutualistic relationship with our microbiota. Those organisms have evolved with us and their genes provide traits that we have not needed to develop on our own. We provide a warm anaerobic, nutrient-rich environment in which they thrive, and in return our microbiota has endowed us with various health effects. It plays an essential role in many body functions. One of the key activities of microbiota is to help us efficiently extract calories from the food we eat (energy harvesting), particularly through fermentation of some carbohydrates that are difficult for us to digest, such as the starch and cellulose found in grains and potatoes. The microbiota is also involved in the production of some vitamins, such as vitamin K and several B vitamins. Our immune system has adapted to tolerate the presence of the normal microbiota; they work together to provide an environment safe from invading infectious agents.

Microbes can eat chemicals, assisting in their degradation. For example, they assist in the breakdown of chemicals in the environment. The gut microbiota in particular can participate in breaking down an abundance of different drugs before they are absorbed. We know very little about the effect of ingested environmental pollutants on the balance of the gut microbiota. We don't know whether ingesting chemicals contributes to overgrowth of bacteria in the intestine or whether eating insecticides can create an imbalance.

More than 90 percent of the intestinal bacteria consist of two types: *Firmicutes* (51 percent) and *Bacteroidetes* (48 percent). These families of bacteria are the same in most of us, but the individual species and strains usually vary from one individual to another; they can be as unique and individualized as a fingerprint. Where do they come from? What would happen if we altered this balance? And what stops the immune system from becoming irritable, given its continuing contact with an over-whelming number of microbials on our surfaces?

C-Sections, Newborn Babies, and the Environment

During its development, an unborn baby is sterile, protected in the uter-us from any microbial exposure until passing through the birth canal to the outside world. The trip down the birth canal immediately exposes the baby to the mother's vaginal, intestinal, and skin flora,[8] all of which are different. Children born by Caesarean section (C-section) are not exposed to the maternal flora in the birth canal, and as a result their ac-cumulating microbiota are different. The intestinal microbiome of infants born via C-section lacks many types of bacteria. In particular, children born by C-section have reduced levels of *Bacteroides* and increased levels of *Staphylococcus*.

They also have pronounced differences in their gut colonization, and these differences seem to persist at least during infancy and per-haps longer. If early establishment of normal intestinal flora is important, could abnormal programming of immune system function be caused by different microbial exposures in newborns after C-section? The short an-swer is yes.

One consequence is infection. Approximately 80 percent of antibiotic-resistant infections observed in infants occur following

---

8 *Flora* refers to the population of microbes in a particular area.

C-section births. Children who were born by C-section are more prone to allergic diseases, particularly the development of food allergies and eczema, as well as asthma. Rates of inflammatory bowel diseases in childhood are also moderately increased; for example, there is an increased risk for Crohn's disease in young boys. Altered immune mechanisms have been associated with the onset of other immune-mediated diseases, such as type 1 diabetes. After normal delivery, cytokine levels are usually low, but they are substantially elevated after C-section, suggesting immune activation. Colonization of the gut with normal microflora is mandatory for proper development of the immune system.

Twenty-five years ago the World Health Organization recommended a C-section rate of not more than 10 to 15 percent in any country. However, for several reasons, including advanced technology to identify infants at risk during labour, recently reported C-section rates are much higher: 25.6 percent in Canada, 30.8 percent in Australia, and 31.1 percent in the United States. So a considerable number of children start their lives with abnormal intestinal environmental exposures and are at risk for abnormal immune system programming and dysfunction.

Differences in the microbial flora in individuals who are born by C-section contribute to immune and inflammatory conditions of the intestinal lining later in life. There is even a suggestion that the incidence of celiac disease is related to C-section. Exposure to antibiotics in infancy may also have long-term negative implications for gut microbial composition.

The Microbiome and Irritable Bowel Syndrome

When ingested food leaves the stomach, it enters the small intestine, which is a 20-foot-long muscular tube, the far end of which joins the large intestine. The purpose of the small intestine is to digest proteins, fats, and carbohydrates and to absorb nutrients before passing the waste material on to the large intestine (colon). The purpose of the five-foot-long large intestine is to reabsorb water from the remaining undigested matter, which is then expelled.

The stomach and the first part of the small intestine normally contain only a small number of bacteria, and one-third of healthy people have no growth at all. We now know that overgrowth of bacteria in the small intestine is more prevalent in irritable bowel syndrome (IBS). Small intestinal bacteria overgrowth (SIBO) occurs when colonic bacteria flow back into the upper intestine; it is present in up to 80 percent of these patients.

SIBO is common in IBS. One reason is that up to 70 percent of IBS patients have co-morbid reflux and gastroesophageal reflux disease (GERD) symptoms, so they frequently use antacids. Frequent use of antacids, especially the proton pump inhibitors (PPIs), promotes the development of SIBO because it changes the environment of the small intestine. While the antacids do reduce stomach acid production, they also have the undesirable side effect of altering the acidity (pH) in the intestine, an environmental change that promotes bacterial growth. Most PPI antacids are sold in pharmacies without prescription; they include omeprazole, lansoprazole, esomeprazole, pantoprazole, and dexlansoprazole.

Besides antacids, there are other factors that can contribute to SIBO. For example, stress can increase the level of the gut bacteria by inhibiting stomach acid release and altering motility. Although we don't yet understand why, SIBO is frequently found in patients with Crohn's disease, chronic pancreatitis, Parkinson's, and scleroderma.

Antibiotic therapy can provide symptomatic improvement in some IBS patients, particularly those with significant bloating. Numerous studies using antibiotics to eradicate SIBO have shown improvement in bowel symptoms, providing evidence that overgrowth of bacteria can be a cause of IBS.

The gastointestinal tract also contains TRPV1 receptors. They detect physical stretching of the intestinal wall and are relevant in many of the processes of digestion. This family of receptors can be sensitized, which is seen in patients with environmentally linked illnesses such as

MCS and fibromyalgia. Both of these groups of patients are more likely to have IBS and GERD. The explanation is, at least in part, changes in the function of these receptors.

Intestinal Permeability

The intestine has a lining that allows for the absorption of necessary nutrients, electrolytes, and water. It also acts as a barrier that selectively prevents harmful substances from penetrating and invading the internal environment of the body. The lining comes into direct contact with high concentrations of bacteria, food antigens, and a multitude of compounds that are potentially toxic or stimulating to the immune system. Its proper function is crucial in ensuring our health and survival.

The intestinal lining is a barrier that consists of two parts. The cells are lined up together tightly so that they do not allow water-soluble substances to go through it. The second component is the spaces between the cells, called tight junctions. Since most water-soluble compounds cannot penetrate the cell membranes, they are transported across the barrier through the surrounding tight junctions. Tight junctions are not static barriers but rather dynamic structures that open and close intermittently. The intestinal barrier membrane is only a single layer of cells that separates the potentially hostile contents of the intestine from the neighbouring tissues of the body. Amazingly, the entire lining is completely renewed approximately every five days.

Oxidative stress can affect some of the structures in the tight junctions, potentially leading to changes in intestinal permeability. Oxidants derived from diet and outside sources constantly challenge the intestinal wall barrier. The microbiome interacts with the lining of the intestinal wall and can also affect the function of the intestinal barrier. Loss of barrier function and increased permeability is known as a leaky gut. When this occurs, there is an effect on the functioning of the immune system and brain. It is linked to the development of allergy and autoimmune diseases such as celiac disease, both type 1 and type 2 diabetes, inflammatory bowel disease, autism, and chronic fatigue syndrome.

The Microbiome, Energy Harvesting, and Obesity

Prehistoric mammals had teeth best suited for eating insects, meat, or fruit. As mammals evolved to consume more plants, they needed the help of intestinal microbes. The addition to the microbiome of bacteria capable of breaking down starch and dietary fibre in the small intestine was important for survival. It enabled herbivores to obtain more calories from the food supply, providing an additional source of energy for the body. Herbivores (plant eaters), carnivores (meat eaters), and omnivores (eaters of both plants and meat) all have a different microbiota.

The composition of the microbiota also differs in lean animals and humans as compared to obese ones. Studies of lean and obese mice indicate that the gut microbiota affects energy balance: it increases the calorie harvest. Obese mice show an increased proportion of Firmicutes and a decrease in Bacteroidetes, and humans show the same results. Interestingly, low-calorie dieting and weight loss increase the Bacteroidetes proportion.

In the laboratory, scientists are able to keep mice sterile, free of microbes; these mice are referred to as "germ-free." In an interesting experiment, researchers discovered that young conventionally reared mice had a 40 percent higher body-fat content as compared to germ-free mice, even though they consumed less food. When they transplanted the intestinal microbiota from the normal mice into the germ-free mice, the latter subsequently developed 60 percent more body fat within two weeks, without any increase in food consumption or obvious differences in energy expenditure. Furthermore, the increase in body fat resulted in insulin resistance and increased levels of glucose in the blood. All these changes occurred because the composition of the gut microbiota affected the amount of energy extracted from the diet.

In a similar study, researchers found that the absence of gut microbiota protected against weight gain in mice that consumed a Western-style high-calorie diet (41 percent fat and 41 percent carbohydrate). The germ-free mice gained significantly less weight than their counterparts that had a normal microbiome. Not only do these studies demonstrate the role of the microbiota in obesity, they also raise the possibility of using gut microbiota manipulation in the treatment of obese individuals, including both the amount and the balance of the flora. More research is needed in this area.

Diet, Gut Microbiota, and Obesity

Like most reactions in the body, the microbiota-diet reaction is bidirectional. The intestinal microbiota has an effect on the energy harvest, and diet has an effect on the quality of the intestinal microbiota. Today we consider the gut microbiota as an organ, dynamic compared to other organs in the human body, because its cellular composition rapidly changes in response to dietary shifts. For example, when we give mice a diet richer in fat, the intestinal microbiota community reacts within 24 hours, resulting in increased levels of Firmicutes. Diet alters the gut microbiota's composition by increasing the levels of Firmicutes, which causes an increase in the energy harvest and results in weight gain.

People who have low levels of Bacteroidetes are more likely to be overweight. Animal studies demonstrate a clear relationship between diet, the microbiome, and weight. Human studies are not as clear, because no matter what the diet (for example, vegetarians versus omnivores), people vary in their eating patterns. Some people only eat at mealtimes, while others snack or even graze continuously throughout the day. Fasting between meals has been shown to increase Bacteroidetes in mice. This implies that snacking between meals, even if it is on healthy food, can make it harder to lose weight or even cause weight gain. It can change the balance of the microbiota.

Children born by C-section, who have lower levels of Bacteroidetes as infants, are more likely to become overweight by age seven. Even preschool children born by C-section are twice as likely to be obese. Similar observations have been made with adolescents. Not surprisingly, a study of several thousand middle-aged adults revealed that those born by C-section were 50 percent more likely to be obese. In a study of overweight adolescents on a diet and exercise weight-loss program, results depended on the quality of the microbiota prior to treatment. The overweight adolescents who lost significant amounts of weight had higher levels of Bacteroidetes prior to starting the program, as well as after.

The balance of the microbiota predicts who is more likely to experience significant weight loss even before that person begins a weight-loss program. Developing therapeutic interventions to manipulate the gut microbiota may be beneficial for weight loss as well as for preventing weight gain. At this point in time the studies to prove this have not been done and the exact bacteria species responsible for the weight gain and weight loss have not been identified. Furthermore, the testing required to accurately analyze the microbiota is not yet routinely available to consumers.

Medications are another environmental xenobiotic source. For example, antibiotics have a significant impact on gut microbes. A five-day course of oral antibiotics modifies the human gut microbiota for up to four weeks. It tends to revert to its original composition, but sometimes it fails to recover, even within six months. The use of antibiotics in infants is associated with a decreased number of anti-obesogenic bacteria such as Bacteroidetes, which may not completely reestablish.

Antibiotics can reduce the overgrowth of intestinal microbiota (SIBO) that is frequently seen in IBS, and many patients get better. But so far no one has looked at whether this treatment influences weight in these patients.

Evidence for the participation of TRPV1 receptors in promoting fat accumulation and body weight is also accumulating. Genetically engineered mice that do not have any TRPV1 receptors will gain significantly less weight on a high-fat diet. Stimulating these receptors may contribute to weight gain. Logic states that we may be at risk because chemical pollutants stimulate these receptors. Could chemical pollution be a factor that leads to obesity?

CHAPTER 13

OBESITY

I guess I don't so much mind being old as I mind being fat and old.

— Benjamin Franklin

In the past 50 years the prevalence of obesity worldwide has increased dramatically, especially in children. The prevalence of childhood obesity has tripled in the past 30 years. In the United States, obesity is now prevalent in more than 30 percent of the adult population. It's not much better in Canada. One in four Canadian adults and almost nine percent of children are obese.

And high-income countries are not the only ones affected by obesity; the condition is rising alarmingly in the developing world as well. The World Health Organization reports that at least one billion adults are overweight and 300 million are obese. And without intervention, these numbers are expected to rise. If the trend continues, the majority of the world's adult population will be either overweight or obese by 2030.

We have already seen that xenobiotics (pharmaceuticals and chemical pollutants) can affect the balance of the microbiota and that this can contribute to weight gain. The environment is involved in the pandemic of obesity in several other ways as well, some obvious and others more subtle. Individuals are blamed when they gain weight and keep it on, but lifestyle is only part of the story. The environment has a huge responsibility in ways that we had never considered until recently.

Earlier I described the biopsychosocial model of medicine, which I adopted in my clinical practice in the 1980s. This model helps to comprehend the total human experience of illness. The environment is also biopsychosocial. *Biology* includes the air we breathe, the food we eat, the water we drink, the ultraviolet radiation from the sun, microbes (including our own microbiome), and so forth. But the environment is also psychosocial. *Psycho* includes the events in your life that affect emotions, such as happiness, anger, or grief. *Social* includes the cultural things over which you have little control but have to adapt to, such as the commute to work, where you can afford to live, recreation and social activities that are available, and even the products that you have grown to depend upon, such as household cleaners and cosmetics. In other words, society influences our behaviours as well.

This biopsychosocial model can be applied to our understanding of obesity. But it is easier to recognize the environment's impact on weight gain by turning the model around and considering it from a social-psycho-biological perspective.

It's Easy to Get Fat, Not So Easy to Be Fat

Anyone can gain weight. There are numerous and more significant causes of obesity beyond an abnormal microbiome. The most obvious reasons are poor eating habits and reduced physical activity because of lack of desire or time, injury, illness, or aging. Other reasons can include taking medication with a side effect of weight gain, or simply moving to a community far enough away to require a longer commute time.

People do not choose to be fat, nor do they want to be at risk for diabetes, coronary artery disease, or cancer. Our culture idealizes thinness and disparages obesity. Most normal-weight individuals are judgmental and attribute obesity in others to simply making poor choices — eating too much, choosing the wrong foods, being lazy. The social consequences of being obese are substantial because of pervasive stigmatization, prejudice, negative stereotyping, and even discrimination. These behaviours occur in several domains, including employment, education, interpersonal relationships, and the media.

Even health professionals are not immune to this anti-fat bias. Medical students describe obese patients as less attractive, more depressed, and less compliant. Family doctors describe these patients as lacking self-control, and one-third of nurses prefer not to care for obese patients at all. The Implicit Association Test is used to measure bias that may not be consciously recognized. When researchers use this test to assess the attitudes of medical obesity specialists, an implicit pro-thin, anti-fat bias is found even in this group.

Why Are We Getting Fat?

Society influences human behaviour. Complex societal factors influence obesity, including physical activity, diet, and the environment. Where you live plays an important role. Do you live in an urban or suburban neighbourhood? How far is it to the corner store, and how much time do you have to go there? How long is your commute to work? Do you prefer to sit or stand when taking public transit? Why is it considered normal to just stand still on an escalator, letting the machine do all the work? Do you have a dog to walk? If you live in a cold climate, do you resist going outside during the winter unless you have to?

Many studies have highlighted the fact that lack of physical activity in our modern Western lifestyle is an obvious contributor to gaining weight. A variety of domestic functions have been automated, such as vehicle transportation and the use of elevators rather than stair climbing. We take numerous labour-saving devices for granted, such as dishwashers, washing machines, and vacuum cleaners. Use of these has been calculated to save us 111 calories per day, and not compensating for this change by reducing food intake could contribute to a weight gain of up to 10 pounds (4.5 kilograms) per year. The increased leisure time available to be physically active is being spent sedentarily, watching television and/ or using the internet and playing computer games.

The Western diet provides many culprits to blame for the epidemic of obesity, starting with tubs of buttered popcorn at the multiplex and fast-food breakfasts that total more than 1,000 calories. Even a trendy *caffe latte* can contain more than 250 calories. Two of these coffees per week can provide enough calories to gain seven pounds in one year (one pound of weight equals 3,500 calories). Although we consume less fat in our diets today, we are eating more energy-dense and processed foods and fewer fruits and vegetables. The growth of the fast-food industry has coincided with the obesity epidemic. Fast foods are low in quality and are energy dense: high in less valuable calories and saturated fats and low in micronutrient content (vitamins and minerals) — and cheap.

Sugar intake is a major source of empty calories, which have no other nutritional value than as an energy source. Sugar was originally a luxury product, accessible only to the privileged classes. But when the price went down about 300 years ago because of increased production in European colonies, sugar became available to everyone. Since the 18th century the rise in consumption of sugar per capita has been closely associated with industrialization, increased personal income, the use of processed foods, and consumption of beverages to which people add sugar, such as tea, coffee, and cocoa. In addition, the popularity of soft drinks has expanded the use of sugar, especially in the form of high-fructose corn syrup. Consumption of this sweetener, which is now used to flavour many prepared foods, from soda pop to breakfast cereals and salad dressings, has skyrocketed since it was developed more than 30 years ago. Consider these statistics: in 1967 Americans ate 114 pounds of sugar and sweeteners per person per year, nearly all of it as either raw or refined sugar. In 2003 each person consumed about 142 pounds of sugar per year. Sugar-sweetened beverages are the primary source of added sugars in the American diet, and they are strongly associated with the rise in obesity, especially in children.

Our social environment and its influence on behaviour can have an impact on whether we gain weight. It can also provide significant stress and emotional pressures. For many reasons it can make us feel anxious, lose sleep, and feel depressed or burned out. Emotional stress can also have a significant impact on weight.

Obesity and the Brain

Many people use "comfort food" to help them cope with stress, anxiety, boredom, loneliness, isolation, abuse, despair, or frustration, because food can provide a biological sense of reward. The connection is not just emotional; it is both physical and mental. The regulation of energy and food intake under stress is biologically linked to survival. So it is not surprising that the limbic system is tightly intertwined with the regulation of appetite. Obese people are more easily stimulated and motivated to eat; the differences in limbic system responses can be measured in functional brain scans. Obese children and adults respond differently, even to pictures of food.

The majority of overweight and obese people in the community are not depressed, but obesity and depression frequently do occur together. Depressed people tend to be inactive and not exercise as much. They tend to eat more, especially comfort foods, because it's harder to be self-disciplined when you're depressed. Taking antidepressants might cause weight gain too, adding fuel to the fire.

Depression can cause weight gain because, when we are depressed, our brains release more cortisol, a major stress hormone. This hormone stimulates and promotes fat storage, especially in the abdomen. But weight gain can also promote depression. We already know that fat releases cytokines, and their effect on the brain includes symptoms of depression. In fact, having higher levels of cytokines can predict its onset.

Following a healthy diet for weight control also reduces the incidence of depression. The relationship between obesity and depression is one more example of a bidirectional communication between organ systems.

There is also a relationship with obesity and sleep. Obesity is an important risk factor for developing sleep apnea in both children and adults. Approximately 40 percent of obese persons have it, and over 70 percent of patients with apnea are obese. Chronic sleep deprivation can also lead to weight gain.

Fat communicates bidirectionally with both the brain and the immune system. The three systems communicate via cytokines. If there is excess fat, the release of cytokines is increased, chronic systemic (whole-body) inflammation is induced, and, on a cellular level, oxidative stress can be triggered or enhanced.

The psychosocial component in our external environment clearly affects our metabolism, and it helps to have that perspective in order to understand obesity. But obesity is a complex condition, and our understanding of it is incomplete without the biological component.

Pollution: Adding Injury to Insult

If you are dieting and exercising to lose weight and getting increasingly frustrated because you aren't dropping as much as you think you should be, it might not be all your fault. Your biological environment might be interfering with the process. The mitochondria are responsible for converting food into energy, but this process is impaired in obesity. The mitochondria become dysfunctional and inefficient. When sensors inside the cells detect that there is less energy available, they communicate with the brain and appetite is stimulated — it makes us want to eat. Mitochondrial function can be affected by oxidative stress caused by environmental chemical exposures, and there is accumulating evidence for the role of pollution in both the rise in obesity and its effect on health.

Animals that live in or around humans in industrialized societies have potential value as canaries in the coal mine too, warning us about environmental factors. Over the past several decades there has been a rise in the average midlife body weights of primates and rodents living in research colonies, as well as in untamed rodents and domestic dogs and cats. These findings suggest that increasing body weight cannot be due solely to chosen lifestyle.

Air pollution exposure has an impact on obesity. Researchers studied the effects of a high-fat diet on two groups of mice. One group was exposed to typical outdoor polluted air and the other was exposed to clean, filtered air. The mice exposed to the polluted air demonstrated more changes. They had higher levels of oxidative stress, more changes in mitochondria, a higher inflammatory response in fat, more insulin resistance, and accelerated atherosclerosis. How does such a thing occur?

The answer can be found in the TRPV1 receptors. The effect of pollution on the receptors is what the canaries have been warning us about. These receptors are found in many areas of the body, and they are also involved in weight control. If we destroy the neurons with TRPV1 receptors in newborn mice, we seem to protect them from diet-induced obesity. How these receptors interact with fat is unclear, but if we turn them off, the mice can eat more fatty foods without gaining weight. If blocking or eliminating TRPV1 receptors helps to lose weight, it stands to reason that stimulating these receptors would result in weight gain. Chemical pollutants sensitize the receptors, which provides a potential explanation of how chemical pollutants are contributing to the development of obesity.

There are other ways in which chemical pollutants contribute to obesity. To understand how this occurs will require some understanding of the biology of fat. Chemical pollutants that we can't eliminate easily, such as persistent organic pollutants (POPs), are stored in fat. In obese people the levels are higher. The more exposed we are to these chemicals, the more weight we gain. If they are just stored in fat, how can they influence our ability to gain weight?

The view that fat is only a passive storage space for unused calories is outdated. Fat is now considered an organ and part of the endocrine or hormone system, because it can secrete hormones and cytokines. In fact, it secretes at least 30 different chemical messengers that play a central role in our metabolism.

Endocrine Disruptors

In the past 20 years evidence has accumulated that a number of pesticides, industrial by-products, and manufactured products such as plastics are endocrine disruptors. In other words, they disrupt the messaging of the hormones that regulate the functioning of many organs. Hormones are the body's messengers, and cells can receive the messages if they have the right receptors. It has to be a perfect fit.

Various pollutants are now being categorized as endocrine disruptors. They have the physical characteristics necessary to fit snugly into the hormone receptors. This phenomenon enables them to interfere with the natural messaging of the endocrine system. The pollutants can mimic or sometimes block the effects of the natural hormones. Even very low doses can stimulate activity.

A link between endocrine-disrupting chemicals and obesity has been proposed for a number of years. In a revolutionary paper published in 2002, the author speculated that obesity cannot be explained solely by alterations in food intake and/or decrease in physical activity, commenting on how the obesity epidemic had coincided with a marked increase of industrial chemicals in the environment. This paper reviewed numerous studies of chemicals, including pesticides, organophosphates, PCBs, polybrominated biphenyls, phthalates, BPA, heavy metals, and some solvents, all of which showed evidence for promoting weight gain. It was suggested that the chemicals could be capable of affecting hormones. Since then, many studies of the effects of low-dose exposures to various pollutants have demonstrated that they can promote weight gain. Chemicals that promote weight gain are referred to as obesogens.

Scientific evidence is mounting that environmental chemical exposures are contributing to the escalating prevalence of obesity. In fact it can start programming changes in our metabolism even before birth. One study exposed pregnant mice to air polluted with diesel exhaust; the level of exposure was typical for humans from outdoor air. When the offspring became adults and were fed a high-fat diet, they gained much more weight than mice that had been exposed to clean, filtered air while in utero. This effect was dramatically more pronounced in the female mice. In humans, studies have shown that higher maternal exposures to ambient air polluted with diesel exhaust or pesticides are associated with childhood obesity. This is caused by a phenomenon known as epigenetics, which will be covered in the next chapter.

The environmental impact on obesity comes from at least three different sources, including hormone-disrupting obesogens, chemicals that activate TRPV1 receptors, and changes in the balance of the microbiome, leading to an increased energy harvest. The fact that xenobiotics can cause unplanned weight gain in humans should not come as a surprise, given that many pharmaceuticals, such as commonly prescribed antidepressants and anti-seizure medications, often cause weight gain as a side effect. Fat is an endocrine organ, and endocrine disruptors can cause havoc in fat.

Overweight Canaries and Systemic Inflammation

Obesity is an environmentally linked illness and has many similarities to ME/CFS and MCS. TRPV1 receptors are involved. People who are overweight are more likely to have ME/CFS and fibromyalgia. They are more likely to have the pattern. They have central nervous system complaints of pain, fatigue, sleep disturbance, and mood disorders such as depression. They are more likely to have respiratory symptoms because of allergies and asthma, and they have gastrointestinal complaints from IBS and GERD. On a cellular level, fat cells in obese people suffer oxidative stress, mitochondrial dysfunction, and impaired mitochondria biogenesis. Exposure to outdoor particulate matter increases the oxidative stress and further reduces the number and function of mitochondria in fat cells.

As we gain weight, fat starts to influence our immune system. Fat cells release messenger cytokines to attract more immune system cells. So the fatter we are, the more they accumulate in our fat. These immune cells also release more cytokines, and together they put people in a state of systemic inflammation.

Obesity is known to be a cause of, or contributor to, many chronic diseases. One reason is that chronic systemic inflammation is a characteristic of obesity. It is important to understand that systemic inflammation is different from acute inflammation. Acute inflammation occurs immediately in response to a perceived attack because the immune system responds to the release of chemical messengers, the cytokines. The cells rush to the area to defend us from invasion or to repair damage after an injury. We have all experienced the classical signs of acute inflammation, which are redness, swelling, heat, and pain.

Systemic inflammation is different because:

☐ it causes only a small rise in cytokines
☐ there are no classical symptoms or signs of inflammation
☐ it has subtle but systemic (whole-body) rather than local effects
☐ it appears to perpetuate rather than resolve a disease.

Obesity is a state of chronic oxidative stress and systemic inflammation. This is why obesity leads to other diseases affected by pollution, such as cardiovascular disease, diabetes, and more.

Health Impacts of Obesity

Health concerns about obesity are not a new phenomenon. Life insurance companies were already using height and weight charts in the 1930s to identify clients who were at increased risk for premature death, in order to adjust their premiums accordingly. Obesity is associated with a number of health conditions. Systematic reviews of the medical literature reveal that being overweight or obese is strongly associated with the incidence of type 2 diabetes, most cancers (excluding esophageal in females, pancreatic, and prostate cancer), high blood pressure, heart disease, asthma, gallbladder disease, osteoarthritis, and chronic back pain.

Obesity is a major cause of metabolic syndrome, which is the term used to describe a group of conditions that often occur together. Each one increases the risk for developing coronary artery disease, stroke, and type 2 diabetes. Metabolic syndrome consists of:

- [ ] insulin resistance (diminished response to normal concentrations of insulin)
- [ ] increased abdominal fat (inside the abdomen, not just under the skin)
- [ ] high blood pressure
- [ ] dyslipidemia, which includes: elevation of total cholesterol, elevation of "bad" cholesterol (low-density lipoprotein, or LDL), elevation of triglyceride concentrations, and decrease in "good" cholesterol (high-density lipoprotein, or HDL).

There are no symptoms associated with metabolic syndrome. You may feel fine, but you are no longer healthy. Having metabolic syndrome means that you are already in the midst of an active disease process. If you are compliant, taking your medications for high blood pressure and high cholesterol, you reduce your risks, but you are still more likely to suffer strokes, heart attacks, and/or diabetes.

Obesity, Insulin Resistance, and Diabetes

One of the components of metabolic syndrome is resistance to insulin. Cells have insulin receptors on their outer membrane to which insulin binds. By attaching to these receptors, insulin allows "doorways" to open. Glucose flows through the doorways and the cells can use the glucose for energy.

When a cell becomes resistant to insulin, the insulin receptors shut down and glucose cannot easily pass through to the inside. Because the cells aren't getting the sugar that they need for energy, this indicates to the pancreas that it has to work harder to produce more insulin. When this happens, measurable levels of insulin in the blood are higher. That is the sign of insulin resistance. When even this elevated level of insulin is no longer effective, sugar levels in the blood remain elevated. That is diabetes. Obesity is the most common cause of insulin resistance. It causes both a decrease in insulin receptors and failure of those receptors to activate.

Oxidative stress is a major cause in the development of insulin resistance. The damage it produces can affect the cell membrane and reduce the number and function of insulin receptors. This leads to a reduced ability of insulin to promote glucose uptake by the cells, leading to diabetes. The link between air pollution and diabetes is explained by these factors.

We also know that obesity contributes to oxidative stress, which in turn leads to reduced mitochondrial number and function and insulin resistance. Numerous studies have demonstrated that obese patients have higher levels of oxidative stress, especially if the fat is abdominal. Gaining more weight will increase the oxidative stress. And because of the oxidative stress, obesity lowers the activity of mitochondria.

The Total Load

One of the theories of environmental medicine that I learned in the early 1980s was the *total load* concept. This was described as the simultaneous effect of multiple environmental exposures on a susceptible individual, each contributing to the breakdown of the body's homeostatic mechanisms. Rarely is only one offending agent responsible for triggering or exacerbating environmental hypersensitivity. The theory was rejected by mainstream medicine at the time.

In April 2012, in an editorial in *Environmental Health Perspectives*, Linda Birnbaum, director of the U.S. National Institute of Environmental Health Sciences (NIEHS) and National Toxicology Program, wrote the following:

> . . . human exposures to thousands of environmental chemicals fall in the range of nonnegligible doses that are thought to be safe from a risk assessment perspective. Yet the ever-increasing data from human biomonitoring and epidemiological studies suggests otherwise . . . [Research has found] low-dose effects for dozens of chemicals across a range of chemical classes, including industrial chemicals, plastic components and plasticizers, pesticides, phytoestrogens, preservatives, surfactants and detergents, flame retardants and sunblock, among others.

The traditional approach of using high doses of toxic substances to predict consequences came from a statement made 500 years ago by Paracelsus, which became a paradigm that toxicologists still use today: "The dose makes the poison." That paradigm did not work to explain multiple chemical sensitivities, and as a result it contributed to the "logical" denial of its existence. The paradigm cannot explain the mechanism of hormone disruptors either. We now know that Paracelsus was wrong. The toxicology mantra should therefore be changed to

> *The dose makes the poison — but there can be more than one poisonous dose.*

If you are one of those people who have tried various diets and exercise but can't get your weight down to normal, do you think the environment might be playing a role? Just consider the multiple pollutant exposures over your lifetime that contributed to repeated hits of oxidative stress, eventually leading to mitochondrial dysfunction. Then add their effects on your TRPV1 receptors. Don't forget to consider the obesogens such as plastics, fire retardants, PCBs, pesticides, and BPA, all of which are present in most people. And there are others, including some chemicals yet to be identified as obesogens. Which one of those pollutants is responsible for your weight problem?

The answer is . . . probably most of them. So if you were born by C-section or are stressed or depressed, can't sleep, don't exercise because you're not motivated or are too busy, eat a typical Western diet and/or are driven by your limbic system to eat comfort foods, you will gain weight, especially if you live in a polluted urban environment, are already overweight, are full of obesogens and endocrine disruptors, and/or have IBS with an imbalanced microbiome. If you attack only one of those parameters, is it any wonder that you can't lose weight? We clearly need a new perspective in our understanding of the prevention and management of obesity.

CHAPTER 14

REDUCTIONISM AND SYSTEMS BIOLOGY

Not everything that counts can be counted, and not everything that can be counted counts.

— Albert Einstein

Western medicine is stuck in a 400-year-old rut. We try to reduce everything we see to its simplest form in order to categorize and label it with a diagnosis. This is reductionism, and we use it to understand what is going on in our patients. The epitome of reductionism in medicine is the Cartesian model, which asks, "Is it physical or mental?" This model has become our culturally specific perspective about disease and is now the dominant folk model of disease in the Western world. For the average person, the emphasis is still on etiology (cause), using the same rigid dualistic frame of reference: it is either physical or it is mental. Because of this, many people have chosen to believe that multiple chemical sensitivities, chronic fatigue syndrome, and fibromyalgia are mental. They do not empathize but instead disbelieve or criticize, and they give advice such as "You need to suck it up," or "You need to get out of your funk." Insurance companies frequently deny disability claims, and physicians often refer these patients to psychiatrists.

Reductionism

The principle of reductionism is the belief that complex systems can be understood by studying their most fundamental parts. If we divide complex problems into smaller, simpler units, we can resolve them. René Descartes developed the concept of reductionism more than four centuries ago. He suggested that the world is similar to a clock, and that we can understand it better by taking it apart and studying the individual components.

Reductionism still pervades medical science and affects the way we diagnose, treat, and prevent diseases. It has been wonderfully successful in acute-care medicine. Examples include emergency appendectomies and the use of antibiotics for bacterial infections. Simple cause, simple cure. What about a coronary angioplasty performed to unblock clogged arteries? That procedure is a miraculous achievement, but shouldn't we also consider the processes that led to the clogged arteries in the first place? After all, they are still ongoing.

We train physicians to practice evidence-based medicine — conscientious and prudent use of the best available evidence to make decisions about the care of individual patients. Undergraduate medical schools teach students to interpret the accuracy, significance, and value of research studies. Evidence-based medicine is now the dominant force in the development of treatment guidelines and controlled studies. Clinical researchers constantly subdivide patients into defined homogeneous groups in order to test who might benefit most from a particular treatment option. This predominant and most valued scientific methodology is absolutely necessary. We need to learn as much as possible in a precise manner.

While we need every new scientific detail to build our understanding of health and disease, clinical application of all these factors requires an understanding of the collective impact on the whole human organism. Reductionism has been responsible for tremendous successes in modern medicine, but it has its limits, and we need to find an alternative methodology to complement it.

Consider the message from the canaries, who say their symptoms are provoked by chemical pollutants that everyone else tolerates. The first response from conventional medicine was incredulity. The doctors were skeptical that the symptoms the patients attributed to chemical exposures could be physical or physiological. This was new, it did not fit the conventional paradigms of toxicity and allergy, and there were no objective measures to confirm its validity. Doctors used reductionism to reduce MCS to a psychiatrically driven false belief, and they discredited physicians who argued against that model.

But the traditional doctors were wrong. We now have objective evidence of a distinct biological entity in the form of abnormal detoxification genotypes, oxidative stress, TRPV1 receptor sensitization, and supportive animal models. However, there is also evidence for an increased likelihood of previous or co-morbid psychiatric illness in MCS, ME/CFS, and fibromyalgia patients. This once again provokes the Cartesian reductionist question: is it physical or mental?

The answer is yes. Yes, because every biological system communicates with all the other systems in a bidirectional — even a multidirectional — manner, from the external environment to molecules inside the cells, even in the brain. They influence the stability or instability of one another. The MCS canaries are not just warning us of the potential dangers of chronic chemical pollutant exposure. They are also telling us to change our cultural, philosophical, and scientific paradigms, which emphasize reductionism to the detriment and exclusion of alternative perspectives.

The primary claim of biological psychiatry is that mental disorders are a form of a physical and/or chemical brain disorder, but clearly the human mind is more than just neurons and neurotransmitter messengers. Considering psychiatric illness only as a chemical imbalance is too simplistic. Patients do not suffer from Prozac deficiency. Looking at the mind as completely separate from any physical or chemical properties of brain functioning (the Cartesian model) is also too simplistic, even naive. The amount of evidence showing biological changes in and outside the brain in psychiatric illness is quite substantial. Chronic psychiatric illness is another example of multisystem dysfunction, and mitochondrial dysfunction and oxidative stress occur in many psychiatric disorders.

Challenges to the Cartesian model began in 1977, when psychiatrist George L. Engel argued that the dominant biomedical model of disease was insufficient for a complete understanding of health. Specifically, he stated that this model "assumes disease to be fully accounted for by deviations from the norm of measurable, biological variables. It leaves no room within its framework for the social, psychological, and behavioural dimensions of illness." Engel advocated that health care needed to integrate the biomedical and psychosocial viewpoints, in what he termed the biopsychosocial model. This model considers not just the body-focused biological components of health but also the individual and societal contexts of the individual's experience of health. It is more closely aligned to the World Health Organization's definition of health: "a state of complete physical, mental, and social well-being and not merely the absence of disease."

The biopsychosocial model is an improvement on reductionism. It recognizes that psychological and social factors influence a patient's perceptions and actions. Therefore this model individualizes the experience of what it feels like to be ill, emphasizing the bidirectional interplay between mind and body. It helps to facilitate our understanding of the impact of an illness or a treatment's effect on the patient's overall quality of life, as well as the impact of resulting psychosocial stressors on the disease process. It has helped physicians and other health care professionals to work together with their patients to deal with the realities of chronic illness and to understand the impact of chronic illness on function and quality of life.

For example, how do we approach the problem when an obese woman, who has always been responsible for feeding her family, is newly diagnosed with diabetes, and she cannot successfully comply with the necessary changes in her diet because the rest of her family does not like the new menu and constantly complains? The biopsychosocial model gives health care providers insight. This biological illness is having an effect on the patient's personal family environment; there is a bidirectional repercussion. Her family's reaction affects her emotionally and she feels that she cannot comply with the treatment. The biopsychosocial model emphasizes that more is required to treat this chronic illness than just prescribing an adjustment of sugar levels.

Although Engel proposed his model in the 1970s, and though medical educational programs have accepted it, its implementation in medical practice is still limited because of the deep-rooted dominance of the biomedical, reductionist model of health. Even our cultural understanding of our physical health is reductionist. Except for trained health care professionals, everyone else is an amateur physician. And everyone uses the same reductionist thinking to understand human biology. Imagine a guest in your home complaining of chest pain. Do you call 911? Perhaps some questions are in order first, such as how long the person has had the pain. If the answer is six months, you are likely to put down the phone.

Third-year medical students are evaluated for their ability to be reductionist. We still ask them the same question I was asked 40 years ago during oral exams: "Imagine you are the emergency room physician and the patient presents with chest pain. What is your differential diagnosis?" Differential diagnosis is the process by which one sifts through the medical evidence to arrive at a final diagnosis. The student must reveal her knowledge and thinking processes clearly as she reviews the potential causes of chest pain. Is the origin of the pain cardiac, respiratory, gastrointestinal, or musculoskeletal? What are the different possible causes of pain from those organ systems? How do they differ? The student must demonstrate not only that she has memorized the list of causes of chest pain but also show an ability to think, to be able to logically sift through that list and establish the most likely causes. She must use reductionism to narrow down the possibilities. She can make the final diagnosis with additional information from the physical examination and appropriate lab tests. The differential diagnostic technique leads to a focused, typically organ-based therapeutic plan, which is very effective in acute-care medicine but is ineffective in the management of chronic illnesses.

Reductionism is prevalent in our culture. In science we use reductionism to attempt to explain complex phenomena. We try to define the functional properties of the individual components of complex systems. Reductionist methods will continue to be an essential element of all biological research efforts, but it is naive to believe that reductionism alone can lead to a complete understanding of how living organisms function and the mechanisms of abnormal chronic, complex medical conditions. With the reductionist approach, we analyze a patient's main complaint by organ system, cellular dysfunction, and/or molecular defect. We often neglect the dynamic interaction of the elements and how they affect the system as a whole. All living organisms are clearly much more than the sum of their parts. We can't understand the behaviour of their complex physiological processes simply by looking at how the individual parts work in isolation.

It might have been acceptable back in the eighties and early nineties for doctors to use a reductionist paradigm to challenge the opinions and practices of physicians who thought outside the box. After all, just because a perspective is new and unconventional is not a guarantee that it is correct. However, those of us who advocated for our patients with functional conditions were also disrespected by colleagues and, indeed, persecuted by some who held positions of power in the politics of medicine. There was no meaningful dialogue, and since that time, most traditional allergists and many toxicologists have remained stuck in the box of reductionist reasoning. And because they are wrong, they have caused significant harm to MCS patients by mislabelling them with incorrect psychiatric diagnoses and testifying as experts against the patients' claims for compensation or disability insurance.

Reductionist reasoning has interfered with our ability to understand the role of the multiple factors involved in the development of chronic disease. In particular, it fails to appreciate the role of constant low-level exposure to numerous pollutants in the development of chronic illnesses.

Many other common conditions are influenced by environmental factors. These include neurodevelopmental disorders in the young, such as attention deficit hyperactivity disorder (ADHD) and autism; neurodegenerative disorders in the elderly, such as Parkinson's and Alzheimer's; obesity; arteriosclerotic diseases such as hypertension, heart disease, and strokes; some cancers; respiratory diseases such as COPD and asthma; allergies; autoimmune diseases; preterm births; and diminished lung development in children. New illnesses that are caused by changes in the environment have emerged, such as chronic fatigue syndrome, numerous chronic pain disorders, and sick building syndrome. Even more frightening is the evidence that chemical exposures and oxidative stress in our unborn children can program increased vulnerability to chronic illnesses later in life, and for subsequent generations. The common denominators of all these conditions are:

- ☐ influence of chemical exposures
- ☐ oxidative stress
- ☐ symptoms of the pattern
- ☐ co-morbidity.

Unfortunately, even if we add the biopsychosocial model to the reductionist model, it is still not enough. The processes underlying the mechanisms of chronic illnesses still continue relentlessly. The illness remains and progresses and we are more likely to develop others. What we need is a paradigm shift and a new model that will enable us to have a better impact on the course of chronic illness.

The opposite of reductionism is holism, which should really be spelled *wholism*, as we can trace this approach back to Aristotle, who said, "The whole is more than the sum of its parts." Who we are as humans is also more than the sum of our parts. Being holistic means looking at the patient and the disease as an entity rather than focusing on interactions at molecular levels. The biopsychosocial approach is holistic, but only if the *bio* component is considered to be multidimensional as well. *Bio* includes genes, chemical messengers, organelles, cells, organs, and systems, plus their interactions with one another and with the external environment. Unfortunately we have devalued the meaning of the term *holistic medicine* by equating it only with alternative/complementary therapies. But the holistic paradigm, which will most likely advance our ability to understand and alleviate chronic illness, is actually systems biology.

Systems Biology and Medicine

The alternative to reductionist reasoning is the systems medicine paradigm. Systems biology directs us to understand the interactions among genes, the systems of cells, tissues, and organs, the external environment, and behaviour. Systems medicine incorporates these complex interactions in order to understand the process of a disease, rather than perceiving the disease as a single abnormal mechanism occurring in isolation and then treating it accordingly.

Here is a simplified diagram of the bidirectional nature of systems biology:

atoms ⇄ molecules ⇄ epigenetics ⇄ genes ⇄ proteins/enzymes ⇄ organelles ⇄ cells ⇄ tissues ⇄ organs ⇄ organism ⇄ emotions ⇄ spirituality ⇄ external biopsychosocial environment

This simple one-dimensional diagram of systems biology illustrates all the interactions from the genes to the environment and back again. But it is still incomplete, because it is an oversimplification. One reason is that the external chemical environment at one end of the diagram does many things simultaneously. It can change internal molecular contents, affect gene functions, or damage organelles, or do all three. The diagram below provides another dimension or perspective. Genes influence genes, chemicals influence chemicals, cells function well because the organelles are in sync, and so forth:

gene ↔ gene

chemical ↔ chemical

organelle ↔ organelle

cell ↔ cell

tissue ↔ tissue

organ ↔ organ

organ system ↔ organ system

human ↔ human

Since each entity in the diagrams can have an impact on any of the others, the best way to provide a dynamic image of all the connections and interactions of living humans would be with a three-dimensional transparent hologram in which you could see all the simultaneous interactions among genes, proteins, organelles, cells, tissues, and organs. But you'll have to use your imagination and create that image in your mind.

Try it now. Concentrate so that you can imagine all the checks and balances in action as every system, from organ to gene, communicates simultaneously with every other. And as you do that, make the image come alive. Observe all the experiences and the subsequent emotional and biochemical responses to the social, physical, and chemical environments. See how they interact with cell function and detoxification systems, influenced simultaneously by mitochondria swimming around the cell producing both the required energy and free radicals. Now put your own face on the image, because that's who and what you are — a constant continuum of all that interactivity, every day, from conception to death.

Homeostasis and Allostasis

Dr. Walter Cannon developed the concept of homeostasis a hundred years ago, demonstrating that the reductionist model was already proving problematic. A Harvard physiologist who also coined the phrase "fight or flight" (the physiological reaction in response to a perceived threat), Cannon declared:

> The coordinated physiological processes which maintain most of the steady states in the organism are so complex and so peculiar to living beings — involving, as they may, the brain and nerves, the heart, lungs, kidneys and spleen, all working cooperatively — that I have suggested a special designation for these states, homeostasis. The word does not imply something set and immobile, a stagnation. It means a condition — a condition which may vary, but which is relatively constant.

Homeostasis, so necessary for survival, is the maintenance of optimal set points, including markers such as blood pressure and blood glucose (sugar). Allostasis is the process of achieving homeostasis. It is the term we use to define all the adaptive processes that actively maintain stability through continuous physiological adjustments or behavioural changes.

The cruise control in your car provides a metaphor for homeostasis, set points, and allostasis. In the early days, cruise controls could not compensate for unexpected forces. The throttle was locked into one speed, but the cruise control could not sense hills (either up or down), wind resistance, or tire pressure. Therefore the car's speed would fluctuate significantly.

The set point was the desired speed, but there were no checks and balances to keep it there. Modern cruise control maintains the steady set point (speed) by continuously monitoring data that its computer registers. The system dynamically compensates for all disturbances — this is allostasis. In this system, if all we observe is the speedometer reading, we will notice very little change. It appears to be a very stable system — homeostasis. We do not see the effects of going up or down-hill, wind gusts, and so on.

Stress

A healthy stress response occurs when an animal appropriately responds to a threat. It involves turning on an allostatic response, dramatically re-setting the set points for heart rate and blood pressure. This is a complex responsive adaptive pathway that shuts off when the threat has passed. At least, it's supposed to.

There are two sides to stress: its adaptive nature and its possible maladaptive consequences. Firefighting is a metaphor for this paradox. Firefighters may use water to extinguish certain fires or even prevent them. But if they use too much water, it can cause more damage than the flames. Another risk is that increased water usage can lead to loss of water pressure, making the firefighting less efficient and contributing to the spread of the fire. Just like the firefighter's water, stress responses are ideally beneficial but can impose a cost on the body. When we call on them too often, or for too long, they don't work as well anymore.

The stress response is controlled by the limbic system. Present in the brains of all mammals, it has the distinct purpose of survival and ad-aptation to the environment. It communicates with the environment by using the cortex, the immune system, and all our senses: light, sound, touch, smell, and taste. It has bidirectional communication with the pre-frontal cortex and the sensory, hormone, autonomic, and immune sys-tems. And it has direct and indirect contact with chemical pollutants.

Allostatic Load

The allostatic load is the price that the body may ultimately pay for its repeated efforts to adapt. It accumulates over a lifetime from exposures to multiple repeated stressors, whether they are emotional, physical, or chemical. It contributes to the normal process of aging. Every time we place a demand on our cells to work harder, we increase the production of metabolic by-products, which need to be detoxified. Repeated hits of oxidative stress are one of the main contributors to the damage caused by the allostatic load. As our pollution exposures have increased, our allostatic chemical load has also increased because of the repeated oxidative stress responses that we endure.

A high allostatic load contributes to cardiovascular, immunological, and neuropsychological disturbances, both acutely and cumulatively over time. Eventually it leads to impaired immunity, atherosclerosis, obesity, osteoporosis, and atrophy of nerve cells in the brain. It affects the limbic system and can lead to increased perception of pain, as well as chronic widespread pain and chronic fatigue syndrome.

Some of the long-term effects of a high allostatic load can be measured, such as changes in blood pressure and heart rate, chronic inflammation, high cholesterol, increased percentage of body fat, elevated sugars, and measurable signs of stress. How many measurable components of the allostatic load do you have?

Allostasis and Systems Biology

The dynamic nature of allostasis helps us to understand the concepts of systems biology. During the past half-century, biological research has revealed how complex biological systems are, especially in humans. An incredible amount of biological data has accumulated, and for that we are indebted to the reductionist scientists. We need them to keep searching to identify even more minuscule, infinitesimal, yet important details of how life works. But now the major challenge is how to understand and use all this data. It is clear that we can't understand this complexity by studying genes and proteins one at a time; we must study biological systems as an integrated whole. Computer technology enables us to do global analysis of many types of information. With this technology, we are also learning how to integrate many different levels of biological information that will help us understand the dynamics of systems.

Systems biology is an interdisciplinary science that has its roots in biology, physics, mathematics, computer science, engineering, and other disciplines. Systems biology integrates computerized technology with applied mathematics, statistics, engineering, biochemistry, biophysics, molecular biology, genetics, ecology, evolution, anatomy, neuroscience, and visualization. The approach is holistic rather than atomistic.

Integrating huge amounts of data in order to study systems is familiar to engineers, for example, those designing control systems for commercial jet airliners. Biologists can learn a lot from the engineers who design these systems, which generate, every minute, a volume of information similar to that in the entire human genome. Building models to understand complex systems is done in other domains as well, such as by meteorologists predicting the path of a hurricane.

Systems Medicine

The practice of medicine can be enhanced by a systems biology approach that would recognize the interactions between all the components responsible for dysfunction of the human system. There are several characteristics of clinical medicine that are fundamentally reductionist. The natural inclination of medical practitioners is to isolate the single factor that is most responsible for the observed abnormality and to treat that factor. Implicit within this practice is the ingrained belief that every disease has a potential single target for medical treatment. For example, the target in infection is the bacteria; for cancer, it is the tumour. The disease, not the whole person biologically participating in and affected by the disease, becomes the central focus.

But in chronic illness a person's sleeping habits, diet, living conditions, age, sex, other co-morbid illnesses, and emotional stress may all have contributed to the onset, continuation, and exacerbation of his or her disease process. Let's look at a heart attack, for example. It is the final result of years of accumulating damage. What about environmental pollutant exposures or the microbiome? They each could have contributed to chronic inflammation, obesity, and oxidative stress — and the evolving cardiovascular disease. What was happening to that patient on a cellular level that eventually led to the heart attack? The oxidative stress from pollution inhaled while driving home from work might just have been the final straw.

Reductionist conventional medicine misuses the concept of homeostasis, treating it as if it were static. We often consider illness as a failure of homeostasis; then physicians try to correct the deviations by driving the parameters back to within their normal range. This corrective treatment approach works for a range of medical conditions from hypothyroidism to diabetes.

Reductionists consider a system as a collection of static components and emphasize static, stable, normal ranges. Their emphasis on correcting a parameter that is outside the normal range disregards the dynamic interactions between parts. Consider hypertension as an example. Using medications to lower blood pressure is good; it reduces the risks for stroke and heart attack. If the medication is effective and the blood pressure remains normal and stable, the correct advice is to keep taking the medication. But the doctors who use this approach are ignoring the processes on the genetic, chemical, and cellular levels that are still ongoing.

Systems medicine evaluates the dynamic states of homeostasis. In the hypertension case we are considering, these are likely still struggling to maintain the status quo, because nothing has been done to fix inadequate checks and balances. They appear to be stable now only because of the effectiveness of the medication. Whatever caused the shift in homeostasis (which in this example is a change in the blood pressure set point) is likely still occurring.

So what? you may ask. Just keep an eye on the blood pressure with regular checkups and adjust or change the medication from time to time accordingly. The answer is this: what the doctors are missing will likely lead to other homeostatic changes and other chronic problems. Doctors should be asking about pollution exposures and giving suggestions about how to mitigate those influences as well. But they don't. This is why most people with a chronic problem eventually end up with more than one.

Do not misinterpret the message. Reductionism is invaluable, extremely beneficial, and absolutely necessary for the practice of good medicine, but it is best suited for acute diseases such as appendicitis or acute exacerbations of chronic illnesses such as asthma. It is also vital as a research tool, providing the details necessary to understand and design systems for research. The problem with reductionism is the assumption that it is the only solution, the only perspective, the only manner in which doctors should think.

Most major universities in Canada, the United States, Europe, and Asia now have education and research departments in systems biology. Its significance as a new paradigm is best emphasized by the Canadian Institutes of Health Research (CIHR), the major federal agency responsible for funding health research in Canada. According to the CIHR's report of a workshop on systems biology approaches:

> It is increasingly recognized that a systems approach to research, in which whole systems can be observed and modified, offers advantages over the historical, reductionist approach of examining individual components of systems in isolation from each other. . . . Modern medicine has evolved to have a predominant emphasis on reductionist science, in which researchers focus on individual components in isolation from the system as a whole. For many diseases this separation of the whole into multiple parts ignores the interactions between these parts and their combined influence in disease pathogenesis. Rarely is an immune or infectious disease process caused by a single modality or failure, but rather by multiple factors acting on many components, either in sequence or simultaneously, to bring

about changes in system-wide behaviour. This is particularly evident for most chronic diseases, including autoimmune diseases such as multiple sclerosis, rheumatoid arthritis, and Type 1 diabetes. . . . Whereas bioinformatics [available biology information] is effective in generating analyses of the parts of a system, systems biology focuses on stringing these parts together to build whole systems and gain an understanding of what happens when things malfunction, such as in disease. . . . Systems biology requires a multi-component integrated program that brings all the necessary areas of expertise together . . . and encourages cross-discipline collaboration.

Chronic illness is about the failure of multiple systems. We could better prevent and treat them if we took a systems medicine approach. We need to look at systems in context in order to understand them; they are more than the sum of their parts. Chronic, often debilitating, sometimes even fatal diseases evolve over time because of the complex interactions and imbalances among the different systems involved.

Taking a Better Look

Most patients with the pattern who come to environmental health clinics are frustrated. Multiple physicians have reassured them that nothing is wrong and that all their lab tests are normal. Yet their quality of life has diminished because of how they feel. Time after time I have heard these patients complain that they are sick and tired of feeling sick and tired. Patients come away from their doctor's office feeling they have been told that it's all in their heads and they should suck it up. They find this demeaning and counterproductive. And they can't just function better on demand. It raises the question that if their complaints are truly valid and significant, why can't we find anything wrong?

There is an old story about a man who one night comes upon an acquaintance on his hands and knees, searching for something under a street lamp. The acquaintance says he is looking for his keys, which he has lost in the nearby park. When the man asks why he isn't looking in the park instead, the acquaintance replies, "Because the light is better over here." Similarly, the physical examination and most laboratory tests available to the clinician examine organ function and look for measurable pathology, because that is where the light is. Where we should be looking in patients with the pattern is inside cells and at cell function, which we can presently do only in a research setting or in a few private labs, at great expense.

These patients have oxidative stress, reduced number and function of mitochondria, and changes in cell membrane receptor activities. This results in altered cell communication and function, with resulting over- and under-reactions by the nervous, immune, and hormone systems. It is analogous to placing three normal young children in the same room to play together, but they all happen to be hungry, irritable, and tired. How long will it take before they are arguing, fighting, and crying? The situation is akin to an unstable psychoneuro-endocrine-immunology system — several wired and tired systems over- and under-reacting to each other, making each other worse with negative consequences.

The whole is greater than the sum of its parts. This truism is how we define the term *synergy*, which is the interaction of two or more agents or forces such that their combined effect is greater than the sum of their individual effects. Sports teams provide an analogy. It doesn't matter how gifted the athletes on a team are; the likelihood of success of any team is based on the teamwork (synergy) of the players, the coaches, and the general manager. Every coach constantly emphasizes the concept that the whole is greater than the sum of its parts. Successful businesses use the same maxim. The complicated human organism is another example of synergy, and all the members of the "human team" have interdependent and significant roles.

Genetics Versus the Environment

When your father's sperm met your mother's egg and you were a single cell, your genetic blueprint was set for life. Every influence after that was environmental. Although many experts argue about how quickly genetic evolution can occur, there is general consensus that very little change in the human genome will occur in just two or three generations (60 years). Genetic transformation and evolution are not contributing to the rapid and significant changes in health patterns that have recently emerged.

Our inherited DNA explains our intrinsic strengths, weaknesses, and predisposition to develop certain illnesses more than others. It is our genetic programming. The environment does not change DNA. We will require many generations for our genes to evolve and adapt to the increased pollution, if such a thing is possible. There has simply not been enough time for the human genome to do so over the past two generations. But what is already being changed by the environment is how the DNA works.

Each of us has genetic strengths and weaknesses that are inherited, passed from one generation to the next. But just because we have a genetic predisposition to develop a disease does not guarantee that we will get it. The genes need to be turned on, or "expressed." One of the factors that can activate genes is the environment. Some individuals have low risk of developing a particular disease as a result of an environmental exposure, whereas others are much more susceptible. For example, there are 13 different cancers associated with cigarette smoking. Smokers don't get them all; rather, they get sick and die according to their individual susceptibilities.

The canaries are another example of genetic vulnerability. They have a genotype that makes them less capable of detoxifying adequately. Until the increase in pollution exposure occurred, their detoxification systems could handle the load. MCS, therefore, was not very common. People who are genetically poor detoxifiers are also more susceptible to the cardiovascular and respiratory effects of air pollution. Having this inherited genetic pattern simply makes these people more susceptible to oxidative stress. But it also takes the chemical pollution exposures to overload their detoxification systems. This intensifies the oxidative stress, leading to subsequent vulnerability to developing MCS or suffering the cardio-respiratory and other ill effects of outdoor air pollution.

Epigenetics

Evolution and changes in DNA take thousands of years, but the evidence that environmental pollutants are actually changing our genetic susceptibility and inheritance is already quite strong. This is clearly a contradiction. How is it possible that changes are taking place before our eyes when they are supposed to take place over thousands of years? The explanation is provided by an area of research called epigenetics. Our DNA is wrapped in a set of proteins called the epigenome. It covers and protects the DNA, but most important, it activates and deactivates individual genes. In 2009 the University of Western Australia announced publication of what they referred to as a complete roadmap of the human epigenome. They described the epigenome as "the clothes that dress a genome," controlling the way genes are packaged and expressed without actually altering the underlying DNA code.

Epigenetics regulates gene expression. During our lifetime, various genes are activated (expressed) or are silent. As a 60-year-old I somehow activated my genes for grey hair, although they were silent when I was 30. Activating or silencing genes occurs by removing their wrappings, modifying the epigenome. The term *epigenetics* is used to describe any process that alters gene activity and expression without actually changing the DNA. It was natural, programmed epigenetic changes that made my hair turn grey.

Now we know that it is our epigenome that ultimately controls whether and when particular genes are expressed. Mounting evidence suggests that inappropriate epigenetic changes and subsequent misinterpretation of the code are linked to numerous diseases, including many forms of cancer and a host of other chronic illnesses. Metaphorically, we had been looking where it was easier to see as we searched for how the environment influences gene behaviours. It appears that genomics is just the tip of the iceberg. The bottom of the iceberg is epigenetics.

We can accurately measure epigenetic changes, and they provide solid evidence of the harm from chemical pollutants. A large number of animal studies provide evidence that supports the role of environmental epigenetics in disease susceptibility. These studies show that there are many agents that can damage an epigenome, including heavy metals, pesticides, diesel exhaust, tobacco smoke, and other environmentally toxic and persistent chemicals.

Pollution Evolution

In December 2009 I attended a four-day workshop given by the Society of Toxicology, a scholarly international organization of toxicologists from academic institutions, government, and industry. The workshop was called "Prenatal Programming and Toxicity II (PPTOX II): Role of Environmental Stressors in the Developmental Origins of Disease." It was the society's second annual conference in this area. The workshop's hypothesis was that exposure to environmental chemicals during the prenatal and early postnatal periods affects gene expression. There were 52 presentations and numerous panel discussions that presented data from both animal and human studies.

I was dumbfounded to learn that very low levels of exposure to chemicals can cause increased vulnerability to disease later in life. I learned that pollutants affect gene expression, and that the resulting epigenetic changes may be an important mechanism for subsequent programmed negative changes.

The presenters were not just a bunch of tree huggers from the animal research community, as cynics might suppose. The impressive list of sponsors for this conference included these organizations:

- ☐ World Health Organization
- ☐ International Union of Toxicology
- ☐ European Environment Agency
- ☐ U.S. National Institute of Environmental Health Sciences
- ☐ U.S. Centers for Disease Control
- ☐ U.S. Agency for Toxic Substances and Disease Registry
- ☐ U.S. Environmental Protection Agency (EPA)
- ☐ U.S. National Cancer Institute
- ☐ U.S. National Institute for Environmental Studies
- ☐ U.S. National Institute for Toxicological Research
- ☐ Eunice Shriver National Institute of Child Health and Human Development.

I was one of only two medical doctors present.

The animal studies discussed repeatedly demonstrated that low doses of endocrine-disrupting chemicals can be toxic, and that two chemicals together, even at doses individually too low to be significant, can be additive and cause changes in the epigenome. Sometimes the effect was not just additive but synergistic.

An editorial in the journal *Reproductive Toxicology* summarized the conference papers and concluded that subtle effects during development can lead to functional deficits and increased disease risk later in life. The risks include male and female reproductive diseases, such as endometriosis and cancers of the prostate, breast, and uterus; obesity; cardiopulmonary diseases; neurobehavioural problems; neurodegenerative diseases, such as Parkinson's; and immune and autoimmune diseases. To me the final bombshell from this conference was the fact that we pass on these epigenetic changes to at least the next four generations. Why is this so alarming? Because, as far as we can tell, the damaged epigenome may not repair itself.

In 2011 the Canadian Environmental Law Association, the Ontario College of Family Physicians, and the Environmental Health Institute of Canada produced another extensive review of the literature. Their main findings were as follows:

- ☐ The in utero and perinatal environment and maternal and early childhood circumstances all play major roles in the risk of later-life disease;
- ☐ There is more and more confirmation for the role of early-life exposures to environmental contaminants in a lifelong vulnerability to chronic disease;
- ☐ The following chronic diseases or conditions are associated with early-life environmental chemical exposures:
  - cardiovascular disease
  - cardiac birth defects
  - low birth weight
  - obesity
  - type 2 diabetes
  - Alzheimer's disease
  - Parkinson's disease
  - developmental neurotoxicity
  - cancer (breast, prostate, testicle)
  - respiratory disease.

We should not be surprised that chemical exposures can cause damage to the epigenome. Damage to the epigenome is caused by oxidative stress. This is pollution evolution.

The Exposome

Complex combinations of genetic, epigenetic, environmental, and lifestyle factors cause most chronic conditions and diseases. The pathways to their development are highly individual because everyone's genome and environmental experiences are unique. Genetics might predict susceptibility, but environmental factors cause 70 to 90 percent of chronic disease risk. The *exposome* is a recent concept that considers everything that is not due to the genome.

We do not yet have the ability to measure the impact of our lifetime chemical and psychosocial exposures from uterus to old age. Developing this ability is essential in order to unravel the major causes of chronic diseases. As we acquire the markers to measure and follow the exposome through life, we will add to our understanding of the complex interplay between the genome, the epigenome, and the environment. The exposome does not just conceptualize the interactions between the environment and the internal biochemistry of life, but reinforces the fact that how we manage the sustainability of our planet's air, water, flora, and fauna is intimately and ultimately linked to the survival, health, and welfare of the human species. When we look at global warming, changing weather systems, the extinction of animal species, and changing human health patterns, it appears that we are doing a poor job.

CHAPTER 15

THE OXIDATIVE STRESS CONTINUUM

If you don't have time to do it right, when will you have time to do it over?
— John Wooden

For 14 chapters, we have explored the various components and reasons for emerging conditions and the explosive increase in chronic illnesses. We have allowed these changes through our hedonistic behaviours and careless management of the environment. In the time since I focused my medical practice solely on environmental medicine, I have evaluated more than 12,000 patients who exhibited a disturbing pattern of chronic conditions. What has become apparent to me is that underlying all of these chronic conditions is a single principle. I call this principle the *oxidative stress continuum*. It is an irreversible but controllable progression from total health to total breakdown, and although we don't have the power to reverse it, we do have the power to be conscious of it, to push back against the many factors propelling it forward, and to modulate or temper its effects.

Breakdown of Health

No one suddenly gets Alzheimer's disease or high blood pressure. Chronic disease progresses slowly, along a continuum that exists even before we are aware of the onset of the disease.

It is oxidative stress that quietly but relentlessly chips away at the molecules inside cells. Eventually there is enough damage to cause a change in cell function. If there are fewer mitochondria, there will not be enough energy for the cell to function properly. If the numbers of mitochondria fall past a critical point, the cells program themselves to die. Neurodegenerative diseases such as Parkinson's and Alzheimer's provide examples of how continuous progressive cell death can propel a disease process forward.

Another place where we see oxidative stress causing damage to molecules is in receptors when they become sensitized. This can make them behave in a sensitive and irritated manner, as occurs in MCS and chronic pain disorders.

Becoming Conscious of Your Continuum

It is of vital importance that you understand the significance of the oxidative stress continuum. What provides the momentum is repeated oxidative stress. You can't feel it and your doctor can't measure it, but you must learn how to counteract it and diminish its effects.

The potential effects of oxidative stress on human health and quality of life range from mild to devastating. MCS patients are highly sensitive to the effects of chemicals. These people — the canaries — serve as an early warning system about oxidative stress, alerting the rest of us to the significance of chronic chemical pollutant exposures. Most of us remain physically unaware that we too are enduring the effects of oxidative stress. This is only because the functional or pathological damage has not yet become apparent.

Today there is no reliable way to screen for oxidative stress damage in clinical laboratories. There are no indications that it is present until something else occurs that might make us aware. Changes in cell and/or organ function should alert us to its existence, but we remain focused on trying to fix the damaged organ instead of looking deeper, into the individual cells. Oxidative stress and changes in organelles alter cell function and can lead to cell death. Oxidative stress occurs in all environmentally related diseases, which so far appear to be both progressive and irreversible.

Oxidative stress is a fact of life. It occurs when we are stressed, when we are fighting off a virus, when our sleep rhythm is disturbed, and when we exercise hard. The medical literature is replete with studies that connect oxidative stress to the natural process of aging — that relentless accumulation of a wide range of unrepaired faults that occurs under normal conditions. We all hope to age in relatively good health, but these days most people face an elevated likelihood of developing a plethora of degenerative conditions and functional impairments. The reason is that chemical exposures also cause and contribute to oxidative stress.

The continuum of oxidative stress affects ranges between little or no change in organelle and cell function at one end and the visible, easily identifiable pathological organ changes of chronic diseases at the other. In the middle of the continuum, between these two extremes, are the patients with only subjective evidence of oxidative stress, which is now causing cell or organ dysfunction without measurable pathology. These patients include those with MCS, ME/CFS, and fibromyalgia.

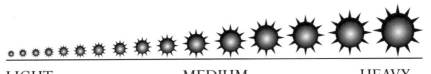

LIGHT
No symptoms

MEDIUM
Functional complaints
Organ dysfunction
No biomarkers

HEAVY
Measurable
organ
pathology

THE OXIDATIVE STRESS CONTINUUM

The oxidative stress continuum is a phenomenon that considers cell health and the ability to detoxify. It weighs the allostatic load and your ability to maintain proper homeostasis set points. With each assault that your cells endure and as the allostatic load increases, the homeostasis of particular systems — molecular, organelle, cellular, and organ — is compromised. The momentum created by this stress moves us all farther along the metaphorical continuum.

This is your life's journey on a cellular level. Starting from conception, the lifelong onslaught of chemical pollutants alters and hastens your journey to the far end of the continuum.

The Middle of the Continuum

In the middle of the continuum are the conditions in which there are only functional complaints, with no abnormalities being found by the doctor. These conditions include ME/CFS, MCS, and fibromyalgia, among others. The link with the environment is oxidative stress.

The cause of ME/CFS is far from clear, but we know that oxidative stress occurs in these patients. This results in reduced number and function of mitochondria, which explains patients' significant fatigue and prolonged recovery after exertion. There is not enough energy production or storage in the cells because oxidative stress is causing damage to the mitochondria. The classical characteristic of fatigue in ME/CFS is that minimal exertion aggravates it. There is simply not enough energy storage. Prolonged recovery time, even after minimal exertion, occurs because the mitochondria cannot replace the energy reserves fast enough. The attempt to exert before recovery increases the oxidative stress. Since oxidative stress plays such an important role in ME/CFS, it is not surprising that many ME/CFS patients also have MCS. This is because oxidative stress is also affecting their TRPV1 receptors. It is obvious that oxidative stress can, and often does, affect more than one location in the cells at the same time.

Patients with ME/CFS and MCS are also more likely to have chronic pain, especially the widespread pain of fibromyalgia, because oxidative stress is involved in chronic pain conditions. This is consistent with the systems biology paradigm: multiple systems are involved, even on a cellular level. Receptors and mitochondria affect each other, with subsequent impacts on cell function. The whole is greater than the sum. As a result, when patients have a combination of ME/CFS, MCS, and fibromyalgia, they are much more functionally disabled.

The Ends of the Continuum

At one end of the oxidative stress continuum is the ability of an organism, whether it is a cell or a complex human being, to maintain normal function and homeostasis. At the opposite end of the continuum is measurable organ damage, consisting of cell death or its opposite — abnormal cell proliferation (cancer).

Oxidative stress has its greatest impact on the cells with the most mitochondria, which are in the brain, immune, and cardiovascular systems. These three systems are involved in most common chronic illnesses and conditions.

Co-morbidity in Chronic Conditions

Chronic diseases are not just becoming increasingly common, they are also linked. Look at the middle range of the oxidative stress continuum. Here we find patients with functional disorders who are more likely to have several, such as ME/CFS, MCS, fibromyalgia, and other chronic conditions such as IBS and chronic pain disorders. They are also more likely to have allergies and asthma. Oxidative stress does not just contribute to the chemical intolerance, fatigue, sleep disturbance, and pain seen in patients with the pattern. It also contributes to the other frequently co-morbid entities such as migraine, osteoarthritis, asthma, chronic hives, and major depressive disorder.

At the far end of the oxidative stress continuum is a wide range of seemingly unrelated chronic conditions and illnesses with measurable pathology, such as neurodegenerative disorders (including dementia, Alzheimer's, and Parkinson's disease), high blood pressure, coronary artery disease, chronic renal failure, and diabetes. And just like the functional disorders, they are all frequently co-morbid. They have underlying mechanisms in common, namely oxidative stress with cumulative mitochondrial damage and dysfunction. And other parts of the cell can be damaged as well.

Endoplasmic Reticulum and Cell Membranes

The endoplasmic reticulum is a network of membranes inside the cells. Its function is to make proteins and to maintain their quality. Proteins are major molecules that perform a variety of functions; they can be enzymes, antibodies, or hormones. They are large molecules made up of combinations of smaller ones called amino acids, which hook together like the cars of a train. But they don't just form one long line; they fold up into particular shapes, which must be perfect in order to function. For example, a hormone is a messenger that must fit perfectly into a receptor on the receiving cell's membrane in order for the message to be perceived by that cell. The endoplasmic reticulum is the cellular organelle responsible for the folding, quality control, and movement of proteins. If it is stressed and does not function properly, abnormal protein folding results.

To produce properly folded proteins and maintain quality control requires an adequate energy supply from the mitochondria. When oxidative stress affects the function of mitochondria, it also contributes to endoplasmic reticulum dysfunction, or even damage. Therefore, environmental disturbances can lead to the production of abnormal proteins.

Properly folded proteins are required for maintenance of the structures in organelles. As a result, endoplasmic reticulum stress and dysfunction can affect the structure and performance of the mitochondria. Once again we find a bidirectional impact (mitochondria ↔ endoplasmic reticulum) with the total effect being greater than the sum. Endoplasmic reticulum stress is involved in chronic inflammation, heart disease, and neurodegenerative diseases.

Lipids are the major component of all membranes. Oxidative stress can damage lipids and change the membrane's structure. If these changes occur in the cell membrane, the outer layer that surrounds the cell, it will make the receptors on the surface more vulnerable to damage. Changing the shape of receptors will affect the cell's ability to receive chemical messages. Brain cells are particularly vulnerable to oxidative stress damage. One reason for this is that neuron membranes are rich in lipids. This helps explain why the brain is the organ most commonly involved in patients with the pattern.

In type 2 diabetes, oxidative stress reduces the function of insulin receptors. However, in MCS, the opposite effect occurs. Instead of reducing their function, oxidative stress sensitizes the TRPV1 receptors, making the neurons irritable and hyperexcitable.

The Pattern, Chronic Diseases, and Detoxification

Is there really an oxidative stress continuum? If so, then patients with functional disorders and oxidative stress should be more likely to develop organ pathology. Thus far very little information is available regarding long-term morbidity and mortality in these patients. CFS patients do have a higher mortality rate; they die earlier from heart failure and cancer. But maybe these patients are at risk just because of their lack of exercise. The results of long-term studies of patients with chronic widespread pain are also contradictory.

What we see in these patients without obvious organ damage is oxidative stress, with effects on mitochondria, cell membranes and receptors, and increased inflammatory messenger (cytokine) production. All the factors that are characteristic of chronic functional conditions such as MCS, ME/CFS, and fibromyalgia are also seen in many common chronic illnesses: increasing prevalence related to pollution exposures, shared risk factors, multi-morbidity, oxidative stress, chronic inflammation, and changes in organelle function. The difference is that we can measure organ pathology.

Our detoxification system has existed for millions of years, but it was not designed to detoxify the hundreds of pollutants to which we are now exposed on a daily basis. Those of us with higher chemical exposures or poorer detoxification systems are even more at risk.

We should heed the warning of the canaries. We are all affected by everyday chemical pollution exposures. Chronic diseases are simply situated further along the oxidative stress continuum.

If you need more evidence that pollution exposure and the burden on the detoxification system is contributing to the increasing prevalence of chronic illness, look what happens to people who are genetically poor detoxifiers but who do not develop MCS, as the canaries did. Poor detoxifiers are more susceptible to the effects of air pollution and are more likely to develop chronic illnesses linked to environmental exposures. In particular, studies show that having that genetic abnormality enhances the risk factors for developing heart disease, increases the risk of asthma and allergy, and makes one more likely to develop chronic progressive neurodegenerative disorders such as Parkinson's, late-onset Alzheimer's, and progressive multiple sclerosis. Being a diabetic and a poor detoxifier increases the likelihood of developing other chronic illnesses such as chronic kidney disease. Oxidative stress contributes to the development of chronic disease, and as our pollution exposures increase, so does the prevalence.

The number of persons in the United States who have multiple co-morbid chronic conditions is large and growing. In 1996 an estimated 99 million people in the U.S. had chronic medical conditions, and 44 percent had more than one. By 2000 those numbers had increased to more than 125 million people. Almost half of all Americans were living with a chronic condition, and the portion of those people with more than one condition had increased to 48 percent. By 2020, as the population continues to age, the number will increase to an estimated 157 million.

In Canada about 80 percent of people over the age of 65 have one chronic medical condition or disease, and approximately 70 percent of those people have two or more. Obviously there is not a sudden automatic deterioration in health on one's 65th birthday. Developing chronic illness is a gradual and insidious change over an extended period of time, involving multiple factors. Clearly, aging contributes to the process of developing chronic illness. In fact it was the study of aging that led to the discovery of oxidative stress. It also emphasized the negative effect of aging on the number and function of mitochondria, now affirmed by thousands of studies.

We are screening and diagnosing chronic conditions with greater frequency and success. This earlier detection means that people can live with chronic conditions and that we can prevent or postpone deterioration or the development of acute events. High blood pressure provides a great example. In one study, almost 700 hypertensive men aged 47 to 55 were followed for more than 30 years. Their blood pressures were well controlled with medication, and for 10 years their health patterns remained the same as for the control group with normal blood pressures. But in the next 10 years the hypertensive men had an increased mortality rate for cardiovascular disease, despite good blood pressure control. During the last decade of the study, their total incidence of stroke doubled, they had 50 percent more heart attacks, mortality from coronary heart disease doubled, and all-cause mortality was increased by a third.

An abundance of studies document the contribution of oxidative stress to high blood pressure. The message from public health programs and your physician is to have your blood pressure checked regularly, and to take medication to control it if it's too high. But that's not enough. The 700 hypertensive men continued to be pushed along the oxidative stress continuum. We need to go further upstream rather than just resetting the abnormal set points of high blood pressure with medication. The prevention and control of chronic diseases would be more effective if we could reduce the number and duration of repeated hits of oxidative stress. The message from the canaries is that we should be doing this even before the development of functional disorders or chronic illness.

Even More Dots to Connect

Where you sit on the oxidative stress continuum depends on your age, genetics, and environmental influences on your body since conception. The older you are, the poorer your natural ability to detoxify oxidants, and the more environmental chemical exposures you have undergone, the more you will have experienced repeated oxidative stress. Being overweight, not exercising, and having had significant psychosocial stress push you even further along the continuum towards chronic illness.

Chronic complex conditions are persistent, substantially disabling, and sometimes life-threatening. They require treatments and interventions across a broad scope of medical, social, and mental health services. Because of the high and increasing prevalence of these disorders, economists and health planners are already questioning the sustainability of our medical and social systems. What is important to the individual is that co-morbid illnesses have an additive — even synergistic — and significantly negative impact on quality of life. The major consequences of multi-morbidity are disability and continuing functional decline, poor quality of life, and high personal health care costs. What compounds the problem is that physicians do not even have guidelines to treat multi-morbidity.

One of the most major and dramatic events in health care was the discovery of antibiotics, thanks to the reductionists. Simple cause, simple solution. But now the most common cause of death and disability is no longer infectious diseases but chronic non-infectious diseases. According to the World Medical Association, whose membership includes most national medical associations, these chronic diseases are not just replacing infectious disease and trauma, they are adding to the total burden of disease in the general population.

Many chronic complex conditions are linked by multiple factors. That is why they are frequently co-morbid. As you move along the oxidative stress continuum, the odds are that you will develop a chronic condition. And then the odds are even higher that you will eventually acquire more.

Cancer

Given the complexity of cancer, it is beyond the scope of this book to address it in much detail. According to the American Centers for Disease Control, cancer is really a group of different diseases. Although each different type of cancer may have its own set of causes, the common denominator is uncontrolled growth and spread of abnormal cells. It is worth noting that, as in other chronic complex diseases, there are links to chemical exposures, obesity, diabetes, sleep disturbance, the microbiome, chronic inflammation, oxidative stress, changes in mitochondria function, and protein misfolding. But instead of the cell dysfunction leading to cell death, the opposite occurs — cell proliferation. The uncontrolled rise in cell reproduction that is characteristic of cancer is opposite to that seen in other chronic illnesses. We do not know what drives oxidative stress to its final pathological destination: cell proliferation or cell death. But we do know that patients with Parkinson's are less likely to develop cancer, because the final pathways of these two diseases diverge in opposite directions.

Common Denominators of Chronic Disease

The following table is a summary of the medical literature. It helps to explain the links between the most common chronic diseases and why they are frequently co-morbid. The headings at the top of the table give the common denominators of the chronic diseases that are listed in the column on the left. All these factors can be caused or exacerbated by pollution, which drives us further down the oxidative stress continuum, increasing our vulnerability and the probability that we will develop another one of these diseases.

Chronic disease	Pollution association	Systemic inflammation	Oxidative stress	Mitochondria dysfunction	TRPV1 receptors	Obesity	Limbic system/central sensitization	Multi-morbidity	Epigenetic Changes
Allergy	√	√	√	√	√	√	√	√	~
Autoimmune diseases	√	√	√		?	?		√	√
Asthma	√	√	√	√	√	√	√	√	~
Chronic obstructive pulmonary disease	√	√	√	√	√	√	√	√	√
Chronic cough	√	√	√		√	√	√	√	
Osteoporosis	√	√	√		√		√	√	√
Chronic kidney disease	√	√	√	√	√	√	√	√	√
Diabetes	√	√	√	√	√	√	√	√	√
Cardiovascular disease	√	√	√	√	√	√	√	√	√
Parkinson's	√	√	√	√	√	√	√	√	~
Alzheimer's	√	√	√	√		√	√	√	~

~ soft evidence √ solid evidence ? early evidence

We all plan to live for a long time, and in good health. Our agenda never includes chronic pain, weakness, and confusion. The oxidative stress continuum is the biological narrative of your life. Pollution simply hastens the pace and alters the course, taking you to places that you never planned to visit. The good news is that you can actively affect that narrative. You have the capacity to change the velocity and direction of the continuum. What you need to know is how.

CHAPTER 16

WOMEN AND CHILDREN FIRST

Eighty percent of canaries are middle-aged women.

— Lynn Marshall

When my son was three years old, he was given a Cabbage Patch Kids doll as a present. This was in the early eighties, when unisex toys were becoming politically correct and trendy. He immediately got down on his hands and knees and drove it around the floor, making noises like a truck.

No matter how hard we try to equalize, males and females are wired differently. We are equal in intelligence but our brains are not identical in structure or function. We process emotions differently and use different neural pathways to do so. We read our social environment differently too. To look at gender more closely, if you travel back up the oxidative stress continuum you will see that women dominate the majority of conditions linked to the environment: MCS, ME/CFS, IBS, and fibromyalgia.

Every workday for the past 27 years, I have seen one middle-aged woman after another. Most are frustrated because their symptoms are chronic, poorly controlled, and not well understood. Their quality of life is diminished, their family members are disappointed and don't understand, and their physicians don't seem to give empathy or support. When psychiatric causes are implied, these patients feel resentful.

Of the 12,000 patients in my practice, 80 percent (or 10,000) are female canaries. Most of them are chemically sensitive. These women are often angry at their employers for not initiating or enforcing scent-free policies, at their colleagues for not following policy requests and disrespecting their sensitivities, and at insurance companies for denying their disability. They are embarrassed by the perception that they are being ridiculed by people who "just don't get it."

Being told that there is nothing biologically wrong and that no one else is complaining, because the usual daily exposures are not toxic, does not help. It's hard to cope when people think you are a complainer and a neurotic, especially because for the first 35 or 40 years of your life you were never like that.

Why is my practice, like every other practice in environmental medicine, dominated by chronically unwell middle-aged women? One reason might be that women report more intense, more numerous, and more frequent bodily symptoms than men, even when gynecological and reproductive symptoms are excluded, and especially when the symptoms are "medically unexplained." Why assume that it's a mental illness? Can that assumption be based on gender bias?

The fact that unconscious, implicit bias can be present in medical professionals has already been reviewed earlier, in chapter 3. Gender bias exists too. For example, critically ill women aged 50 years and older are less likely than critically ill men to be admitted to an intensive care unit (ICU) and to receive potentially life-saving interventions. They are also more likely to die in the ICU or in hospital. Several studies have shown that women are less likely than men to be referred for invasive cardiac procedures.

The POWER of Women

Women are more likely to use health care services. Is that why more females are seen in environmental health clinics — because they show up and complain more? The POWER Study (Project for an Ontario Women's

Health Evidence-based Report Card) is an ongoing comprehensive study of women's health. This research provides the most current evidence on women's health status, their access to health services, the quality of the care they receive, and the outcomes of that care. Its report states that significant health inequities are associated with gender, income, education, and ethnicity.

One chapter of the report is devoted to chronic illness. As reported in many other studies, Ontarians of lower socioeconomic status experience much higher levels of chronic disease and disability than those who are more advantaged. They are also more likely to die prematurely. Women are more likely to be in these lower socioeconomic groups. They are also more likely to report co-morbidity (multiple chronic conditions) and disability than men. The burden of chronic illness and disability is highest among low-income and aboriginal women.

The POWER study acknowledged the environment as a determinant of health eight times in the report's chapter on chronic illness. But it never addressed why or how. It did not address the environment as a more significant issue for females — but it clearly should.

Sex, Gender, and the Environment

The environment does have a greater effect on women. For example, the effects of persistent organic pollutants on high blood pressure are greater in women. The prevalence of metabolic syndrome has increased by 23 percent in women, compared to just 2.2 percent in men, and the incidence of asthma is much higher in women and is increasing. When we examine the effect of air pollution on respiratory health, there are differences between women and men: more studies report stronger effects among the former.

Sex is a biological construct. *Gender* is a social construct that includes cultural norms, roles, and behaviours. It affects where people spend their time and what activities they perform, thereby influencing their exposure to pollutants.

The biological differences between men and women reflect how we respond to the environment. Men have significantly higher systolic blood pressure at rest and higher elevations with stress, while women have a significantly higher heart rate at rest, which increases with stress. Losing a spouse has a greater effect on men with heart disease than on women with heart disease. Is this difference biological or social?

There are sex differences in how the limbic system responds. Functional brain scans reveal that men and women activate different parts of the limbic system after the same stimulation. There are sensory differences as well. On average, women are more sensitive to pain and have a higher prevalence of pain-related conditions. They also tend to have a heightened inflammatory response compared to men.

Women and Chemicals

Much of our information about how the human body handles chemicals has come from the pharmaceutical industry, because of the importance of understanding how we absorb, distribute, metabolize, and eliminate medications. We know that at least 70 percent of adverse reactions occur in women, and the reasons for this unfortunate difference have to do, at least in part, with how women handle chemicals biologically, compared to men.

First of all, normal kidney clearance of chemicals is lower in females compared to males. There are two phases of detoxification, which were described in chapter 7. Detoxification of xenobiotics is usually faster in men. One particular system, which is often involved in Phase 1 detoxification, is slower in women. This means that women can experience a buildup of intermediate metabolites, which can be even more toxic.

Finally, compared to men, women have a higher percentage of body fat at all ages, which can affect the distribution of chemicals that are not easily eradicated. In other words, women have more "cupboard space" for storage of chemicals that are fat-soluble. People who are obese retain more inhaled chemical pollutants. Because women have a higher percentage of body fat, they retain more inhaled volatile organic compounds than men. There is evidence, gleaned from the American *National Health and Nutrition Examination Survey (NHANES)* studies, that women have higher levels of chemicals from plastic (specifically BPA) than men.

Gender and Environmental Exposures

Women who have low-status jobs as well as complex responsibilities outside the workplace quadruple their risk for coronary artery disease. And when women who work at the same occupational level as men go home, their blood pressures and heart rates remain elevated, while men's decrease. This difference is likely because women continue to have more responsibility at home and less relaxation time. Given their greater domestic responsibilities relative to men, women experience more exposure to chemical cleaners, detergents, and fabric softeners. Women also use more cosmetic, skin care, and scented products.

Women are more sensitive to their environment via both the limbic and immune systems. They have a greater body burden of chemical exposures and less efficient detoxification systems, compared to men. So when we travel along the oxidative stress continuum, it is not surprising to find that the patients with chronic illnesses but without measurable organ damage are mostly women. This includes irritable bowel syndrome, chronic pain disorders such as fibromyalgia, chronic fatigue syndrome, and multiple chemical sensitivities.

Women have more chemical exposures and are less capable of eliminating them. They also have the sole responsibility of protecting their unborn children from toxins. The developing fetus is exposed to low doses of several hundred chemical pollutants, coming from both its mother's stored xenobiotic burden and her daily exposures. Every unborn child is at risk for negative effects on its development during periods of vulnerability that can impact its future health, including increased susceptibility to chronic illness as an adult.

More research is required, but we should all be uncomfortable blindly accepting the reassurance from the American Chemical Council that "levels of man-made and natural compounds detected in Americans remain low." If a study were designed in which the xenobiotic burden was lowered in order to observe for long-term health benefits, which study group would you want to be in — treatment or placebo?

Children

Children are more vulnerable to the effects of chemicals because they have greater exposures relative to adults, immature detoxification systems, and still-maturing organ systems. Children's exposures to environmental contaminants are higher than in adults because of the way children interact with their environment. Kids eat with their hands, infants explore things by putting them in their mouths, and both play on the floor (including dusty carpets) and use plastic toys. They also have a higher metabolic rate, meaning that, relative to their size, they eat, drink, and breathe more than adults.

Pulmonary function tests measure how well the lungs take in and release air and how well they move gases such as oxygen from the atmosphere into the body's circulation. Lung function normally increases as children grow in size; this is referred to as lung function growth. Multiple studies show adverse effects of long-term exposure to urban air pollution on the expected growth of lung function development in children of all ages. The more time kids spend outdoors and the closer they live to major roadways, the more likely they are to have reduced lung function growth by age 18. Even preschoolers can be affected: prenatal exposure to fine particulate matter makes it more likely to happen in early childhood.

It should come as no surprise that kids with a genetic predisposition to poor detoxification are more likely to have their pulmonary function growth affected by air pollution. Exposure to air pollution increases the rate of allergies. Children living in urban areas are more allergic, compared to those from rural areas. Numerous studies demonstrate the increased likelihood of wheezing, asthma, and allergic rhinitis in kids who experience more exposure to outdoor air pollution.

There has been a significant rise in chronic complex conditions in childhood. Presently one child in six is being diagnosed with a developmental disability — the prevalence has increased by 17 percent over the past decade.

Childhood Obesity

Childhood obesity is another chronic condition that is increasing at an alarming rate. In the United States, the prevalence of obesity among children and adolescents has doubled during the past 20 years and tripled in the past 30. More than one-third of children aged two to 19 are overweight, and more than 10 percent are obese. Along with these increases in rates of pediatric obesity are startling observations that the prevalence of obesity is increasing for children aged two to five, and even for infants and toddlers. What makes these figures even more alarming is that childhood obesity has significant potential to become a lifelong health problem. Over 50 percent of obese children and 70 to 80 percent of obese adolescents will become obese adults, with the accompanying increased risk of developing cardiovascular disease, diabetes, and other chronic disorders. Puberty can even kick-start the onset of obesity in kids who are merely overweight.

Both oxidative stress and systemic inflammation are present in obese children. At the onset of obesity, there are no co-morbidities. However, with the increase in childhood obesity comes an associated rise in the incidence of both type 1 and type 2 diabetes in children, which are rising at a startling rate. Data from a study funded by the Centers for Disease Control and Prevention and the National Institutes of Health were released at a meeting of the American Diabetes Association in June

2012. The study revealed that there has been an increase of 23 percent in type 1 diabetes and 21 percent in type 2 diabetes among children and adolescents in the past eight years.

Type 1 diabetes is an autoimmune disease that usually occurs before the age of 20. People with type 1 diabetes are usually thin. However, now we are seeing a significant rise in type 1 in obese children, even under the age of five. In type 1 diabetes the immune system attacks and destroys the cells in the pancreas that produce insulin. In type 2 diabetes we see resistance to insulin, rather than pancreatic destruction. There appears to be an autoimmune process happening in obese children. Astonishingly, if the statistics for increased BMI in children don't change, the lifetime risk of type 2 diabetes is estimated at roughly one in three for males and two in five for females for all children born since 2000. As a result, some epidemiologists now predict that the rising life expectancy will level off or even begin to decline within the next 50 years.

An imbalance in energy intake and expenditure appears to be the obvious cause of pediatric obesity, just as it is in adult obesity. But it is hard to attribute lack of exercise to the rise of obesity in infants and toddlers. Obesity is also a multifactorial condition, with a number of underlying biological, social, genetic, and environmental determinants. One of the environmental factors in early childhood that can predict the likelihood of developing obesity is the quality of the microbiome in early childhood. Breastfeeding plays a positive role in developing a normal balance of intestinal flora and is associated correspondingly with a decreased likelihood for obesity. Cow's-milk formula and cow's milk are associated with greater weight, length, and weight-for-length, all beginning in the third month of life.

Oxidative stress occurs in childhood obesity and diabetes just as it does in adults. We also see oxidative stress in abnormalities associated with both low and high birth weight, which can lead to obesity in childhood. There is also a direct correlation between oxidative stress and other childhood systemic diseases, such as non-alcoholic fatty liver disease, growth hormone deficiency, asthma, and juvenile idiopathic arthritis. And let us not forget the prenatal exposures to obesogens.

Autistic Spectrum Disorder

What about autism? Reported rates of autism increased tenfold from the 1970s to the 1990s, and now approximately 1 in 88 children has an autistic spectrum disorder. The numbers continue to climb. Many people differ over whether the observed increase in autism over the past two decades is, in fact, real. Some claim that the increased rates are an illusion brought about by more heightened awareness of the disorder, changes in definitions, better access to services for diagnosis, and/or manipulation by parents seeking increasingly available funding and services for their challenged children.

It is difficult to determine scientifically whether these claims have any validity and, if they do, how much they actually contribute to the changing statistics. Reviews that have downplayed the rising trend have been roundly criticized for their poor methodologies. The evidence supporting an increasing rate for autism has gathered strength. According to the U.S. Centers for Disease Control (CDC), this increased prevalence among American children should be considered an urgent public health concern.

The psychiatric fraternity has chosen to narrow the criteria for the diagnosis of autism, which will have the effect of lowering the prevalence and temporarily diminishing our ability to accurately observe changes in rates.

Autism and the Environment

There are more than 3,000 high-production-volume chemicals out there. Fewer than half of them have been tested for their potential human toxicity, and less than 20 percent have been tested for their potential to cause neurodevelopmental toxicity.

According to the American Academy of Pediatrics (AAP), research indicates potential harm to children's health from a range of chemical substances. The AAP Council on Environmental Health has recently recommended revision of the chemical management policy in the United States to emphasize protection of children and pregnant women. Toxic substances have the capacity to disrupt the development of any of the body's organ systems. The nature and severity of that disruption depend upon the type of substance and the level and duration of exposure. What is most important is the timing of the exposure during the developmental process. This is known as the window of vulnerability. The developing brain is uniquely and exquisitely susceptible to permanent impairment from exposure to environmental substances, especially during those timed windows. This vulnerability is greatest during embryonic and fetal life, especially in the first trimester of pregnancy.

Autism spectrum disorders affect behaviours that emerge at a stage when children usually become increasingly social and communicative. The underlying anatomical changes found in the brains of people with autism likely develop prior to birth, long before the symptoms become apparent. Environmental exposures during the prenatal and early postnatal periods can interrupt normal brain development and cause behavioural abnormalities and cognitive deficits that may not manifest until later in life. There is evidence that this is playing a significant role in the development of autism.

Air pollution exposure during pregnancy can have physical and developmental effects on the fetus. For example, maternal exposure during pregnancy to the by-products of fuel burning, such as polycyclic aromatic hydrocarbons (produced by the burning of diesel fuel), is associated with impaired brain function and developmentally delayed cognition. These same pollutants also have a direct negative effect on one of the genes identified as a risk for autism.

Several studies have associated autism and prenatal and early life exposure to air pollution from traffic. It should concern us all that 28 percent of childcare centres are within 200 metres of a major highway. One small study of children whose mothers lived near well-defined sites of agricultural organochlorine pesticide application, while they were pregnant, showed an increased incidence of autism. Autism also appears to be related to living closer to power plants, which emit many pollutants, including mercury, a known neurotoxin.

Other Factors in Autism

Autism usually becomes apparent after routine vaccination for measles, mumps, and rubella (MMR). A mercury-containing substance called thimerosal was used in the MMR vaccine, and many studies have attempted to link thimerosal to autism. But autism cases have continued to increase since the removal of thimerosal from the vaccine.

The disorder is not related to childhood vaccinations; this is a misconception. The U.S. Institute of Medicine and the World Health Organization have done extensive literature reviews to validate this. The onset of autism after receiving a vaccination appears to be only a coincidence in time. Autism becomes apparent at the stage when a child should be developing communication and social interaction skills but cannot. The damage from the environment occurred much earlier.

There is some evidence for a genetic component to autism, but it can account for only a small fraction of cases. Given that the prevalence cannot be explained by genetics alone, logic dictates that the cause must be environmental, although the search for a single environmental cause has been frustrating. If the environment is having a major impact on the autism spectrum, one should find evidence for oxidative stress, epigenetic changes, and organelle (mitochondria) dysfunction, even when no single environmental factor can be blamed.

Children with autism show a decreased ability to detoxify and an elevated body burden of xenobiotics. Numerous studies have demonstrated that oxidative stress plays a pivotal role in the development and clinical manifestations of the autistic spectrum. When oxidative stress is initiated by environmental factors in vulnerable individuals, it can lead to epigenetic changes that are found in autism. Clearly the abnormal behavioural and cognitive features that define the autism spectrum arise from dysfunction of the brain, and we do find mitochondrial dysfunction in the brain areas responsible for the disorder.

The Pattern in Autism

There is abundant evidence for the pattern in autism: obvious limbic system involvement caused by damage, immune dysfunction, gastrointestinal disturbance, and inflammation. There is also some evidence for impaired carbohydrate digestion, imbalance of the microbiome, and increased prevalence of obesity. And young adults with autism have increased rates of dyslipidemia and high blood pressure.

We need to carry out more studies. We need to compare the health and neurodevelopment of babies conceived and developed in women who have a high body burden of xenobiotics to those who have a lower burden. We are all relentlessly exposed to chemical pollutants from conception to death, and how we cope biologically with this onslaught depends on our gene pool, epigenetic changes, the functioning of our systems for detoxification, our socioeconomic level, and the lifestyle choices that we make: where we live, what we eat, and whether or not we smoke or exercise.

We can influence some of these risk factors by making better choices, but some cannot be altered. We cannot help being children when we are very young, we have no say in our gender at birth, and getting old is something we all hope to achieve. The older we are, the longer our exposures, and the more significant our exposome becomes, the further we travel along the oxidative stress continuum.

PART V

WHAT YOU CAN DO

NAME_____ AGE_____
ADDRESS_____ DATE_____

☐ LABEL
REFILL 0 1 2 3 4 5

_____
(SIGNATURE)

CHAPTER 17

THE NINE-POINT PLAN

Most specialists tend to think in silos. They don't want to hear about anything other than their specialty. I had so many appointments I felt like a major loser. Like all I do is go to appointments. I felt like no one was listening to my whole story with the idea that it may all be linked together.

— F.T., patient

Navigating the Maze of Medical Treatment

All clinical practice guidelines and disease management programs focus on one condition. Yet co-morbidity and multi-morbidity are so common, we ought to consider them the norm in chronic illness.

F.T. is a 46-year-old woman who came to see me because she had chronic fatigue and fibromyalgia. She also had the other central nervous system complaints seen in the pattern: she had sleep apnea, was anxious and depressed, and complained of poor concentration and distractibility. Also consistent with the pattern, she had gastrointestinal complaints from irritable bowel syndrome and reflux, and respiratory complaints due to chronic asthma. Not surprisingly, her immune system was dysfunctional too. She had recurrent bronchitis, numerous bouts of pneumonia, and frequent vaginal yeast infections. She also had inhalant, food, and multiple drug allergies and had been diagnosed with polycystic ovarian disease, which is an autoimmune disorder.

F.T.'s limbic system was clearly hypervigilant. She was sensitive to the odours of multiple chemicals, and contributing to the hypervigilance was a childhood history of bullying and abuse. Furthermore, she was very obese and diabetic, with high blood pressure and elevated cholesterol levels. She was taking 14 different medications prescribed by numerous physicians. Although it can't be measured clinically, she had oxidative stress, systemic inflammation, reduced number and function of mito-chondria, and central sensitization. She was already well advanced along the oxidative stress continuum.

Various specialists had addressed F.T.'s problems from a reduction-ist point of view, but clearly a systems medicine approach is required to treat patients like her. Unfortunately, people with multiple chronic conditions are particularly vulnerable to receiving poor-quality medical care. They tend to use more medical services, which makes coordination of care more difficult. The doctors work in isolation and communicate with each other only occasionally, usually by letter. It is the patients who are ultimately responsible for their own care. As the number of their health care providers increases, patients are likely to find it more chal-lenging to understand, remember, and reconcile the different instruc-tions of those providers.

Of F.T.'s 14 prescribed medications, three have the side effect of weight gain. Because patients with more than one chronic condition usu-ally require more medications, they are also more likely to suffer adverse drug events. Sometimes a treatment for one condition cannot be used in another. For example, drugs called beta blockers are frequently used for heart disease, but they can exacerbate lung problems in patients with asth-ma. Having multiple chronic conditions also makes it more challenging for patients to participate effectively in their own care, because fragmented medical care from a variety of health professionals makes it difficult to or-ganize information and adhere to instructions. Conflicting advice can range from treatment, management, and medication to exercise and diet.

Complex patients require more time and effort to achieve a good level of care, which creates special challenges in communication. They have more to discuss with their primary physician, resulting in less time being spent on each topic, since the duration of appointments remains fixed. Not surprisingly, patients with multi-morbidity rate their doctors lower in patient–doctor communication.

Studies show that these complex patients perceive both their physical and emotional quality of life as poor, regardless of their age. Compounding these issues is the distress they feel when they try to get information about their particular combination of chronic conditions. Sadly, as of yet there are no guidelines for the care of multi-morbidity. All of this adds to the frustrating negative experience of having multiple chronic illnesses. This is reality for these patients.

The U.S. Institute of Medicine's 2001 report *Crossing the Quality Chasm* highlights the problem of compartmentalizing each condition and stresses the need for better continuity of care and integration of services. Realigning the focus of health care and research to be more in line with the complex experience of patients is central to developing solutions that work.

When we look at complex chronic medical conditions from the systems medicine perspective, patterns emerge. Whether there are objective, measurable changes (such as in cardiovascular diseases) or none (as in chronic widespread pain), multiple systems are involved. And in all these conditions we find chronic inflammation, oxidative stress, and negative changes in organelle number and function, most commonly in the mitochondria. Any approach to preventing or treating multi-morbidity must consider these common denominators. The goals of treatment should include slowing down the progression of each illness and improving patient function and quality of life, both physical and emotional. Unfortunately, most treatments for chronic illnesses do not halt progression.

How to Stop It

What you need whether you have one chronic condition or multi-morbidity — or you simply don't want to develop any — is to halt the slide along the oxidative stress continuum. The ultimate goal is a comprehensive program that stops the oxidative stress, repairs and increases the number of mitochondria, improves cell function, reduces inflammation, reduces disability, increases physical functioning, reduces negative emotions, and enhances quality of life while reducing mortality.

Such a comprehensive program was actually invented by my grandmother, who told me when I was a little boy that I needed plenty of exercise, but outside, in the fresh air and sunshine. She told me that I had to keep my room clean, eat all my vegetables, take my daily teaspoon of cod-liver oil, and go to bed without a fuss when it was bedtime. No excuses were tolerated. And she always told me that she loved me.

Born before the invention of the airplane, my grandmother died at the age of 94. She had never heard of oxidative stress. However, since that time I have been to medical school, practised environmental medicine for 30 years, seen more than 12,000 patients with the pattern, and reviewed thousands of published studies, most of which support the information in this book. These experiences give me licence to expand upon my grandmother's highly successful nine-point program for good health and longevity — or in other words, for oxidative stress management:

1. plenty of exercise
2. fresh air
3. a clean room
4. sunshine
5. plenty of sleep
6. vegetables
7. cod-liver oil
8. no excuses
9. feeling loved

1. Plenty of Exercise

Are you in good shape? For the past two decades, assessment of the fitness of Canadians has relied almost exclusively on the body mass index (BMI), a number that we can easily calculate from height and weight. You can search for "BMI calculator" on the internet and calculate yours. However, it is limited as an assessment of overall fitness, because it is only one marker. For example, the BMI is only an approximate measurement of percentage of body fat, and it does not indicate how much fat is visceral (abdominal). To measure overall fitness, one should also consider muscle strength, endurance, cardio-respiratory fitness, blood pressure, blood lipids, glucose tolerance, and insulin sensitivity.

The Canadian Health Measures Survey is the most comprehensive direct health-measurement survey ever conducted in Canada. The survey collected key information from 5,600 people by means of direct physical measurement of such factors as blood pressure, height, weight, fat indicators (waist circumference, thickness of skin folds), and physical fitness testing. The results were appalling. Forty-one percent of Canadian adults had a high total cholesterol level. In the group aged 20 to 39 — the supposed peak period of health — only 27 percent of males and 23 percent of females achieved "excellent" or "very good" aerobic fitness ratings. At 60 to 69 years, 10 percent of males and less than 5 percent of females had excellent or very good ratings for aerobic fitness. How fit are you?

Americans are even worse off, according to a collaborative survey performed by both Statistics Canada and the U.S. National Center for Health Statistics. Compared to Canadians, American adults are 24 percent more likely to be overweight or obese, 59 percent more likely to be inactive during leisure time, 19 percent more likely to report no or low active means of transportation such as walking or biking, and 39 percent more likely to have all those sedentary markers. Obese Americans are 90 percent more likely to be inactive during leisure time, 41 percent more likely to report no or low active transportation, and 73 percent more likely to report all the sedentary markers. Approximately 70 percent of Americans are not regularly active during their leisure time. Worse yet, 25 percent are not active at all. Only 15 percent participate in activities of sufficient intensity, duration, and frequency to improve or maintain cardio-respiratory fitness, and 50 percent of those who do start an exercise program drop out during the first six to 12 months.

It is unlikely that anyone who has got this far into this book doesn't know that exercise is good for them and helps to control or reduce weight. So why am I addressing it now? Because, consistent with the systems medicine paradigm, exercise has multiple effects on several systems: organ, cellular, and molecular. During aerobic exercise, the muscles require an increase in available oxygen. When the pulse and respiratory rate go up in response to this increased demand, there is an upsurge in the supply of oxygen to all cells, including the brain cells. The most obvious effect is on the endocrine system: we lose weight with exercise. On a molecular level, it reduces oxidative stress. Exercise training favourably alters lipid metabolism, increasing the amount of HDL ("good cholesterol") molecules. And the impact on the cardiovascular system is obvious: medically prescribed and supervised exercise can reduce mortality rates of persons with coronary artery disease. From a biopsychosocial perspective, exercise can have a positive impact on symptoms of mood disorders such as depression and anxiety, even when they are associated with menopause.

On a cellular level, with respect to messaging, exercise training has an important effect on insulin sensitivity. Furthermore, aerobic exercise has an immune system effect. Each session of exercise induces an anti-inflammatory environment, and long-term exercise training reduces the level of inflammatory messengers. But most important is the effect of exercise on mitochondria reproduction. Endurance exercise increases the number of mitochondria. Both endurance exercise and low-volume, high-intensity training (such as short bursts of intense resistance exercises with machines or free weights) will increase mitochondrial size and number. A cell cannot make more mitochondria after being damaged by oxidative stress, but an increased oxygen supply can induce the remaining healthy mitochondria to reproduce. Exercise training is thus a useful (and inexpensive) intervention for many degenerative diseases in which mitochondria dynamics plays a key role.

From an environmental perspective, physical exercise mobilizes fat. This means that fat cells release lipids into the bloodstream for energy. It also mobilizes stored pollutants, which should assist in reducing the total body burden.

Assuming that you do not have cardiac or respiratory failure, your arterial blood is saturated with oxygen. The only way you can increase the supply of oxygen and drive it into the cells to stimulate and encourage mitochondrial health is by aerobic exercise. Although you can't increase the amount of oxygen in your bloodstream, you can increase its rate of delivery. Given that there are 1,440 minutes in every day, surely you can find 30 in which to exercise?

2. Fresh Air

Where do you get fresh air these days? Unless you live in a rural environment and you're not too affected by regional pollution, getting fresh — meaning clean — air is difficult. We know that there are health effects when the air pollution is higher than usual, but we don't know the safe levels for any of the outdoor pollutants in the long term. What is more disturbing is the fact that we spend 90 percent of our time indoors and, especially with respect to volatile and semi-volatile organic compounds, our exposures are higher indoors.

The studies of people who live closer to traffic repeatedly demonstrate increased risk for cardiovascular disease, asthma, allergies, and preterm births. How close are you to the nearest busy street (defined as 10,000 cars per day)? You can obtain that information from your municipality. So, how do you get fresh air?

3. A Clean Room

How can you clean the air in your house? Should you open the windows to get "fresh" air? Which is worse, the polluted air outside or the contaminated air in your house? If you increase the ventilation, how can you clean the air coming into your house? Can you reduce indoor sources of contamination?

4. Sunshine

Sunlight can be bad for you. Ultraviolet rays from the sun, which penetrate the atmosphere more easily since we thinned out the ozone layer, can cause skin cancers. But sunshine also activates vitamin D. We need vitamin D for calcium and bone metabolism, it may offer protection against the development of type 1 diabetes, and it may help protect against some cancers, such as breast and colon.

Sunlight also has a positive effect on the limbic system. It is necessary to refine the circadian rhythms of the brain and for maintaining a proper sleep/wake cycle and other hormone rhythms. And, as a Canadian, I can tell you how nice the warmth of the sun feels. Should we be using heat from the sun as a treatment?

5. Plenty of Sleep

No one listened to my grandmother, and now insufficient sleep is endemic. Self-reported sleep duration has decreased significantly since the 1970s. Sleep disturbances, including sleep deprivation, sleep apnea, and shift work, may lead to the development of insulin resistance, obesity, and high blood pressure, all components of metabolic syndrome. Today more than 30 percent of adult men and women between the ages of 30 and 64 report sleeping less than six hours per night. At the other extreme, sleeping more than eight hours per day is also associated with increased morbidity and mortality. Sleeping the proper amount at the proper time — to be in synch with the sun and circadian rhythms — is important.

6. Vegetables

In 1969 researchers discovered an enzyme that breaks down oxidants, preventing damage to cells. The concepts of oxidative stress and the importance of antioxidants came much later. Since the best and most important source of dietary antioxidants is vegetables, I wonder whether my grandmother was psychic.

7. Cod-Liver Oil

As a child I was required to take a teaspoon of cod-liver oil every morning. Somehow my grandmother intuitively knew about the importance of fish oils and the vitamins found in extracts from liver. The oil may be an important source of antioxidants, but it still tasted disgusting.

8. No Excuses

My siblings and I had to swallow that cod-liver oil. We had to eat our vegetables and go to bed at a decent hour. We even had to go outside to play in the winter. No excuses. But now we can eat whatever we want, whenever we feel like it; we can stay up as late as we like; and even if we are overweight and unfit, we can use whatever excuses we want to not change our behaviour. The most common excuse is "I don't have time," but I am sure you have others, such as "I hate exercise," "I can't live without meat," or "It's too hard." Why do intelligent, educated people who are overweight and sedentary, and maybe even smoke, listen to their doctor's warnings that they must change and reply, "I know," with a sheepish grin — yet still not change? How would you explain that to my grandmother?

9. Feeling Loved

There is no question that people who feel good about themselves and who have good social support have better statistics for reduced morbidity and mortality. Spirituality and religion help too. And cultivating positive changes in the limbic system by practising meditation is also beneficial.

A Treatment Program

To reduce or reverse the cellular erosion caused by oxidative stress, we have to convert the wisdom of my grandmother into a treatment program and apply it by using the systems medicine paradigm. None of the individual components of her program is very effective on its own, but each one has an additive or synergistic effect on the others. Imagine if you implemented all nine parts of the program. You could lower your xenobiotic body burden to take the pressure off your detoxification system. You could protect yourself from those relentless exposures to pollution. And you could stop the destruction of your mitochondria and encourage them to regenerate.

CHAPTER 18

TAKE A LOAD OFF

You can wait forever for perfect conditions or you can make the best of what you've got now.

— Jack Layton

There are two requirements for lowering the pollutant load on the body's detoxification systems: (1) decrease consumption and intake of pollutants, and (2) dissipate and deplete what is already stored. Most consumers are familiar with the term *shelf life*, which describes how long a product will last before it deteriorates. In chemistry we use the term *half-life* to describe how long it takes for a substance to decrease or diminish by one-half.

Some pollutants have a very short half-life: they degrade into something else quite rapidly. Other pollutants are quite resistant to degradation and break down slowly. These persistent organic pollutants (POPs) accumulate in the environment, especially in the fatty tissues of living organisms, and make their way into the food chain. The food chain consists of plants that produce food, herbivores (plant-eaters) that eat plants, and carnivores (meat-eaters) that eat the herbivores, plus smaller carnivores. The food chain is actually a pyramid. There are many more plants than herbivores, and even fewer carnivores. Humans sit at the top of the pyramid. We eat everything, and POPs from all the levels below us end up accumulating in our bodies.

Most of the inhaled volatile organic compounds (VOCs) from indoor air have short half-lives in humans — in the order of minutes to hours for the first elimination phase — and leave the body within days. Unfortunately, we keep inhaling them. We see the same thing from exposures to plastics. For example, bisphenol A (BPA) has a short half-life: four to five hours. Elimination should be virtually complete within 24 hours, yet it is measurable in more than 90 percent of the population because of our almost constant exposures. The primary source of BPA is food, but it has also been measured in recycled and carbonless copy paper, dental sealants, dust, air, sewage effluents, and leachate from landfills.

To assess environmental exposures, we can approximate the levels by monitoring our air, food, and water. Measuring what is in our body at any given time would provide a more accurate view of the body burden, but that is highly expensive and is just a snapshot of the moment. For the purpose of assessing sources of exposures, environmental physicians take an environmental exposure history.

One key to slowing or stopping your voyage along the continuum is to understand the extent of your xenobiotic exposures. These are factors you can control; you have the ability to limit them. Simply becoming conscious of the chemicals around you will make you want to change your lifestyle. It will change your perception, your buying habits, and your life decisions.

Environments in Your Life

The following section examines your exposures by dividing them according to various environments. While the lists may seem extensive, they are actually far from complete. As you go through them, notice the environments that are relevant to your life and see how many of the points you recognize as villains that threaten your own well-being. Just like an environmental physician, you need to take a good history.

The environmental exposure history is summarized by the mnemonic CH2OPD2, which stands for Community, Home, Hobbies, Occupation, Personal Habits, Diet, and Drugs. This has been used in a series of papers published in the *Canadian Medical Association Journal* (*CMAJ*) to address various specific exposures.

Community

- ☐ Is the community rural, urban, or suburban?
- ☐ Is the community regionally contaminated?
- ☐ Is the neighbourhood near environmental contamination?
- ☐ Is the community close to industry?

Home

- ☐ How close is the home to a major thoroughfare or highway?
- ☐ Is the home a house or an apartment? Apartments tend to have negative pressure to increase ventilation, which may contribute to contamination from neighbours, such as tobacco smoke. Basement apartments are more likely to have increased mould exposures.
- ☐ How old is the home? Houses built between 1950 and 1970 often have asbestos installed as a spray-on material. Asbestos that is in good condition and not respirable is generally not a risk. However, when it becomes frayed or crumbles, asbestos fibres can be released into the air.
- ☐ What are the sources of indoor air pollution? Examples include smoking, cleaning products, off-gassing of new materials, fire retardants, stain repellents, candles, and personal care products.
- ☐ Is there a gas stove? Gas stoves can cause high levels of nitrogen dioxide, and particulate matter and VOCs increase as well.
- ☐ Is there an attached garage?

☐ Have there been recent renovations? Building materials, home improvement products, and textiles used in the home can pose health risks. For example, formaldehyde is given off by particle-board, insulation materials, carpet adhesives, and other house-hold products. This is a particular problem in the confined spaces of mobile homes. Dust from old paint, either from stripping or peeling, may be a source of lead.

☐ Which common household products are used? These include cleaners, deodorizers, and a host of other products.

☐ Are pesticides and lawn-care products used? Carpet dust levels correspond to the application of pesticides, both indoors and outdoors. Pesticide use indoors, using routine professional crack-and-crevice application, creates measurable levels for up to two weeks after application. Accumulation is seen on furniture and toys because of redistribution, even though they are not directly sprayed.

☐ Are there recreational hazards? Unsealed pressure-treated wooden playground structures may allow children skin contact with potentially hazardous wood preservatives, including arsenic compounds, pentachlorophenol, and creosote. People who frequently eat at pressure-treated picnic tables, or play on or work with them, may also be exposed.

☐ What is the source of water? Municipal water is treated with fluorides. Private wells can be a source of pollutant exposure, especially for industrial solvents, heavy metals, pesticides, and fertilizers.

☐ Are there any adults in the home who may have occupational exposures? If so, are their clothes laundered at home?

☐ What is the basement like? A crawlspace, a dirt floor, or an ineffective sump pump can increase humidity and contribute to levels of microbial growth such as moulds and bacteria, as can a history of water damage.

Hobbies

- ☐ furniture repair (solvents, dust, paint)
- ☐ welding (manganese)
- ☐ painting or arts and crafts (solvents, glue)
- ☐ stained glass (lead)
- ☐ jewellery making (heavy metals, glue)
- ☐ woodworking (solvents, glue)
- ☐ gardening (pesticides, fertilizers)
- ☐ model building (solvents, glue)

Occupation

- ☐ Do you commute a long distance to work? How do you travel?
- ☐ Where do you work? There is a difference in exposures between industrial and non-industrial workplaces. The important elements of the environmental exposure history in the non-industrial workplace include mechanically ventilated sealed building, recent renovations, loading docks, indoor garage, community, and proximity to photocopying.
- ☐ What type of job do you have? Significant chemical exposures can occur in shops that sell carpets or perfumed products, in hair and nail salons, and so on.
- ☐ Do you know your rights? In the industrial workplace you can request details of any chemical exposures. The Canadian Hazardous Products Act is the foundation for the workers' right-to-know legislation enacted in every province and territory, and Canada's national hazard-communication standard, the Workplace Hazardous Materials Information System (WHMIS), includes provision of material safety data sheets (MSDSs). Similar legislation exists in the United States.

Personal

- ☐ Do you use cosmetics and/or perfumed products?
- ☐ Do you have a lifetime history of smoking, excessive use of alcohol, or use of street drugs?
- ☐ Do you go to tanning salons?
- ☐ Do you apply pesticides on your body or clothing (for example, when camping or hunting)?

Drugs

- ☐ Do you take medications? Most medications can have effects on enzyme systems for detoxification. Repeated use of antibiotics and antacids can contribute to flora imbalance of the microbiome.
- ☐ Do you use homeopathic remedies? (heavy metals)
- ☐ Do you take Chinese herbal medicines and/or other botanical supplements? (heavy metals, pesticides)

Diet

- ☐ How much and what kind of fish do you eat? Some fish, such as swordfish, shark, tuna, and marlin, are more contaminated with mercury than others. Fish from new hydroelectric reservoirs may be contaminated by pollutants leaching from the soil.
- ☐ Do you eat food containing additives? There are many food additives, such as artificial food colouring, flavourings, and so on. Artificial dyes derived from petroleum are found in thousands of foods. In particular, breakfast cereals, candies, snacks, beverages, vitamins, and other products aimed at children are coloured with dyes.
- ☐ How much farmed meat and fish do you eat? What about the pesticides used to produce animal feed? How many contaminants does the cow eat before we eat the cow?

☐ How is the food you eat packaged? The major source of plastic found in almost everybody is food contamination. BPA, which is present in the lining of food cans, is an endocrine-disrupting chemical. Polyfluoroalkyl chemicals (PFCs) are used widely in consumer products to make them resistant to stains, oil, and water. In particular they are used in food packaging. PFCs are also endocrine-disrupting chemicals.

☐ How many helpings of vegetables do you eat per day?

☐ How many helpings of fruit do you eat per day?

☐ Do you eat foods with added sugars (e.g., fructose, glucose, sucrose, high-fructose corn syrup)?

Reduce Exposures

After reviewing your exposure history, how can you reduce your exposures? They are, after all, in your air, your food, and your water.

Check the Air Quality Index, or the Air Quality Health Index, if it's available. You can leave the city at least temporarily, on weekends and holidays, to spend time outdoors. At the very minimum, even choosing to avoid major traffic areas can help. In a study of asthmatic pedestrians in London, England, less measurable inflammation and reduction of lung function was found after they walked around Hyde Park for two hours than after walking along Oxford Street, where they were exposed to more traffic fumes. When you consider moving to your next home, consider its proximity to major traffic. But, since 90 percent of our time is spent indoors, it is likely more effective to clean your indoor environment.

You can improve the indoor environment by reducing your levels of indoor contamination. Identify the sources listed above. You can remove chemicals and paints stored in the home. Stop using scented products, including air fresheners, laundry detergents and fabric softeners, toiletries, and cosmetics.

You can improve the indoor air quality further by increasing ventilation and filtering the air coming in from outside. The most energy-efficient way to do so is with an air exchanger, a heat-recovery ventilation system, and a filter. In an air exchanger, one fan blows the stale, polluted air out of the house while another replaces it with outdoor air. Of course, if the outdoor air is cold, you need to warm it up. To do so in an inexpensive, energy-efficient manner, a heat-recovery ventilation system uses the heat in the outgoing stale air to warm up the fresh air. It can also help cool the air in the summer. The best filter to reduce particulate matter from the outdoor air is a high-efficiency particulate air (HEPA) filter.

But reducing our contamination exposure is not enough. We have to take more of the load off.

CHAPTER 19

DIET AND DETOX

Life expectancy would grow by leaps and bounds if green vegetables smelled as good as bacon.

— Doug Larson

Diet is where we have the most environmental control but the least self-control. It is not just a source of contamination, it also a source of calories and nutrients. Eating organically grown foods and meat from animals that are fed a vegetarian, preferably organic diet can enhance reduction of chemical exposures. Fish that are smaller and lower on the food chain, that are not bottom-feeders like shellfish, and that are caught wild, rather than farmed, are all less likely to be contaminated.

Gaining Weight

Diet is especially significant if you are overweight or obese. Calorie restriction is mandatory, not just to lose some weight but to achieve a BMI close to 21, which is just below the midpoint of normal (the range of normal is 18.5 to 24.9). My experience with patients is that most of them have not had a BMI of 21 since they graduated from high school. Given that we lose muscle mass as we age, our BMI should not be going up.

The environmental contributions to weight gain are obesogens, maternal influences before birth, and an altered microbiome contributing to the energy harvest. Psychosocial stress contributes to the bad choices we make. But mostly it is specific dietary and other lifestyle behaviours and choices we make that affect the success of the eat-less-and-exercise-more strategy for preventing or reversing long-term weight gain.

Weight gain often occurs gradually over decades, making it difficult for most people to perceive the specific causes. A 20-year study was done of 120,877 American women and men who were free of chronic diseases and not obese at the beginning of the study. The researchers were looking for changes in lifestyle factors and associated weight changes. Most participants gained an average of 3.35 pounds every four years. It was not surprising to see an association with intake of potato chips (adding 1.69 pounds), potatoes (1.28 pounds), and sugar-sweetened beverages (1 pound), but the study authors were surprised to find gain in weight also associated with red meats (0.95 pound) and processed meats (0.93 pound). At the other extreme, weight loss was associated with an increased intake of vegetables (a reduction of 0.22 pound), whole grains (0.37 pound), fruits (0.49 pound), nuts (0.57 pound), and yogurt (0.82 pound).

The average height of American women is 5 feet 4.6 inches (164.1 centimetres). Assuming that an average woman had the ideal BMI (21) when she graduated from high school, she would weigh 125 pounds. If she were an average person in the above study, her BMI would be in the overweight category by the time she was 46. And this does not take into account factors such as poor sleep, lack of exercise, and the effect of obesogens, including medications. If she gained only two pounds per year, she would be officially obese by age 45.

Clearly the first thing to do to stop gaining weight is to cut out the empty calories. Many diets tout their success with weight loss, but there can be biological costs. Just losing weight is not necessarily healthy if it is done in an unhealthy fashion.

People have different metabolisms. Some people gain weight more easily than others. Someone with a high metabolic rate is able to burn more calories. An individual with a slower metabolism doesn't use as many calories, so the extra available calories are saved and then converted to fat. Aging and being sedentary decrease our metabolism, contribute to an impaired ability to regulate energy balance, and induce weight gain. One key to this metabolic difference is that obese people have a lower capacity for the mitochondria to convert oxygen into energy. The metabolic rate is related to the ability of mitochondria to bind and use oxygen to create energy. The greater the mitochondrial ability to do so, the higher the metabolic rate will be, which means the body expends more energy. Whether this is a cause of obesity or an effect of it is not known, but people with a higher metabolism don't gain weight as easily as others.

When we compare various weight-loss diets, the results can depend on the parameters being measured. Reduced-calorie diets result in clinically meaningful weight loss regardless of which macronutrients they emphasize, carbohydrates, fats, or protein. Weight change is greater in those who adhere most closely to the program, regardless of the type of diet being followed. The choice of diet should include other goals besides weight loss, such as reduction of oxidative stress and avoidance of xenobiotics. For example, the Mediterranean diet, which emphasizes foods lower on the food chain, has better results for reducing oxidative stress and insulin resistance when compared to a low-carbohydrate diet.

Let's consider the goals of the recommended treatment. Overweight people must lose weight to reduce their oxidative stress and chronic inflammation effects. They must detoxify to reduce the xenobiotic body burden, including endocrine disruptors and obesogens. They need to reverse the damage caused by oxidative stress and to increase the number and function of mitochondria.

Vegetarian Diets and the Oxidative Stress Continuum

Vegetarian diets are beneficial in the prevention and treatment of certain diseases such as cardiovascular disease, hypertension, diabetes, and cancer. The evidence is strong that diet is a key environmental factor affecting one's progress along the oxidative stress continuum. The amount of oxidative stress in young women aged 20 to 30 does not differ between vegetarians and non-vegetarians, but there is a marked difference between these two groups as they age. By ages 60 to 70, vegetarians have less body fat, lower cholesterol levels, higher antioxidant levels, and less evidence of oxidative stress than non-vegetarians.

Our exposures to chemical pollutants start at conception. Prospective mothers should note that vegetarian mothers secrete substantially fewer xenobiotic substances in their breast milk, compared to non-vegetarian mothers.

What About Protein?

Many people are concerned that they will become protein deficient if they follow a vegetarian or vegan diet, a fear likely based on the incorrect assumption that the only sources of protein are meat, dairy, and eggs. But you don't need to eat meat to get protein.

Protein is made from amino acids joined together in a chain. We can get all the essential amino acids we need by eating a variety of beans, grains, nuts, and seeds. According to the Academy of Nutrition and Dietetics, which is the largest organization of food and nutrition experts in the world, vegetarian diets are nutrient-dense and consistent with dietary guidelines, and they recommend them as a choice for weight management because they do not compromise diet quality.

In the past, vegetarian diets were described as being deficient in several nutrients, including protein, iron, zinc, calcium, vitamins A and B_{12}, omega-3 fatty acids, and iodine. Numerous studies have since demonstrated that the observed deficiencies were usually due to poor meal planning. It is the position of the American Dietetic Association that appropriately planned vegetarian diets, including total vegetarian or vegan diets, are healthy and nutritionally adequate and provide health benefits in the prevention and treatment of certain diseases. Vegetarian diets are appropriate for all stages of the life cycle, including children, adolescents, pregnant and lactating women, and the elderly. And, despite claims by some critics, there is no substantial evidence that vegetarians are at risk for osteoporosis and bone fracture. Although a vegetarian diet can meet the current recommendations for all the above nutrients, the use of supplements can provide extra protection against deficiency.

The Paleolithic Diet

When a vegan diet is recommended to patients, some are enthusiastic while others won't even consider it. One option for those who feel that they cannot do without meat is the Paleolithic diet. This diet is also referred to as the caveman, Stone Age, or hunter-gatherer diet. It consists of foods that are assumed to have been eaten by humans prior to the development of agriculture, a time known as the Paleolithic period. It began approximately 2.5 million years ago, when humans first started to use stone tools, and ended with the emergence of farming approximately 10,000 years ago.

Although the human genome has remained largely unchanged during the past 10,000 years, our diet and lifestyle have become progressively more divergent from those of our ancient ancestors. These changes began with the dawn of the agricultural revolution and have been accelerating in the past half-century. We may be citizens of the 21st century, but genetically we are still hunter-gatherers from the Paleolithic era.

The principal components of the Paleolithic diet are wild animal foods, such as lean meats, fish, and eggs, and uncultivated plant foods, including vegetables, fruits, roots, and nuts. The diet excludes grains, legumes, dairy products, salt, refined fat and sugar, and processed oils, all of which were unavailable before humans began cultivating plants and domesticating animals. While this was the way we ate before the agricultural revolution, these foods now provide only about one-quarter of the caloric intake of the average European or North American. Now we get most of our energy from grains, dairy products, refined fat and sugar, and legumes.

The Paleolithic diet is increasingly acknowledged as a healthy option because very low rates of cardiovascular disease and diabetes have been observed to correspond with it. There are reductions in blood pressure, lipid levels, and insulin resistance, and the intake of antioxidants is higher compared to the modern Western diet. While both vegan and Paleolithic diets increase the intake of antioxidants, a major difference between them is the protein sources. The vegan diet provides all the essential amino acids to make protein from nuts, seeds, grains, and beans. The Paleolithic diet derives its protein from meat and fish.

The meat must be lean. Until the 1940s, cattle ate grass in pastures. Now high-energy grains are fed to cattle to improve the efficiency of beef production, by decreasing days on feed and increasing the amount of marbling (intramuscular fat). Grass-fed or pasture-raised beef is lean. It has lower fat and cholesterol content when compared to grain-fed beef, and the omega-3 fatty acid levels are higher.

Vegan Versus Paleolithic

An argument against the Paleolithic diet is that meat consumption, particularly of red and processed meats, is generally perceived to be unhealthy; eating meat is correlated with cardiovascular mortality and other chronic diseases such as cancer of the colon and lung. Eating meat increases the chances of being diabetic, and even more so if one eats processed meats, such as sandwich meat, sausage, hot dogs, bacon, pepperoni, and red meat in frozen entrées. Fish is also a source of contaminants with higher levels of heavy metal contamination such as mercury; environmental hormone-disruptor levels are higher in fish-eaters than vegetarians.

Since animals are higher in the food chain than plants, the level of xenobiotics is increased in the sources of animal protein. Add to this the fact that antioxidants are absent in meat. Compare the amount of calories in an eight-ounce steak to half a pound of salad. The steak contains 385 to 440 calories, depending on the cut — equivalent to eating five pounds of romaine lettuce! Pound for pound, meat is more calorie-dense and nutrient-sparse than vegetables. Perhaps a better approach would be to reduce the intake of meat, as in the Mediterranean diet, or eliminate it completely, as in a vegetarian or vegan diet. To lose weight in a healthy manner, eat foods that are calorie-sparse but nutrient-dense.

Many health professionals have encouraged people to reduce their intake of red meat, even though it is an excellent dietary source of iron and zinc and the main source of vitamin B_{12}. Scientific evidence is accumulating that meat itself is not a risk factor for Western lifestyle diseases; the risk comes from the excessive fat, and particularly the saturated fat, found in the meat of modern domesticated animals. To follow the Paleolithic diet properly, one should eat wild game animals or at least lean meats, if they are farmed. In comparison with domesticated animals, wild game animals have a consistently lower fat content. And fat is where the xenobiotics are stored. To reduce the sources of xenobiotics in your diet, farmed animals should be range-grown and organically fed, and fish should be small (lower on the food chain) and caught wild. Or don't eat them at all.

An argument in favour of the vegan diet is that vegetable protein may provide better protection from heart disease than animal protein. There is also less fat in a vegan diet. A six-ounce broiled porterhouse steak contains about 40 grams of protein, but it also contains about 38 grams of fat, 14 of them saturated. The same amount of salmon gives you 34 grams of protein and 18 grams of fat, but only 4 of them are saturated. Meanwhile, a cup of cooked lentils has 18 grams of protein and less than 1 gram of fat. So when it comes to saturated fats, the lentils are the healthiest.

The Mediterranean Diet

The Mediterranean diet consists mostly of fruit, vegetables, whole grains, legumes, seeds, and olive oil. Fish and seafood are recommended to be eaten frequently, and chicken, eggs, cheese, and yogurt with moderate frequency. Meats and sweets are considered only occasional additions to the diet. With its emphasis on fruit and vegetables, this diet is rich in antioxidants. It gained much recognition and worldwide interest in the 1990s as a model for healthy eating habits and disease-preventing characteristics. Its popularity has continued to increase among both the general public and the scientific community.

Research has shown that the Mediterranean diet tends to be more effective than low-fat diets and appears to induce long-term changes in the risk factors for cardiovascular disease, inflammatory markers, and cancer. New data suggest that it may also prevent cognitive decline and risk of dementia.

Although people tend to lose weight when adhering to this diet, the vegan diet, which eliminates the fish, chicken, eggs, and dairy products, promotes more weight loss and greater corresponding health benefits.

Eating Healthy

The medical literature is quite clear that the classic Western diet is the most unhealthy way to eat, because of its excessive sugars, empty calories, extra fats and oils, excess salt, and low fibre content. It is also full of chemical additives.

The increased intake of refined sugar in the Western world during the past 50 years has been reviewed earlier in this book (see chapter 13). In particular, the consumption of high-fructose corn syrup has risen dramatically, contributing to weight gain and imbalance of intestinal flora. Refined sugars are essentially devoid of any vitamin or mineral content. They should be eliminated from your diet as much as possible.

Sugar is not the only source of excessive yet empty calorie intake. Over the past century there has been a 130 percent increase in per capita consumption of salad and cooking oils, increased consumption of shortening by 136 percent, and an increase in margarine consumption by 410 percent. Manufacturing procedures alter the characteristics of vegetable oils. Margarine and shortening are produced by solidifying or partially solidifying vegetable oils via a process called hydrogenation. This process produces saturated and trans fatty acids that are rarely found in natural human foods, and the Western diet frequently contains excessive amounts. The large-scale addition of refined vegetable oils to our diet has significantly altered both the quantity and quality of fat intake.

The daily requirement for sodium (salt) of healthy adults is only 1,500 milligrams. The average dietary sodium intake in Canada and the United States is more than twice that, at approximately 3,400 milligrams per day. About 75 percent of that intake comes from salt added to processed foods by manufacturers; 15 percent comes from personal use (cooking and table salt use), and the remaining 10 percent occurs naturally in basic foodstuffs. In other words, 90 percent of the salt in the typical Western diet is added.

Refined sugars, vegetable oils, dairy products, and alcohol are devoid of fibre. Furthermore, 85 percent of the grains consumed in the United States are refined and, as a result, fibre-depleted. Whole grains contain 400 percent more fibre than refined grains. Even better sources of fibre are fresh fruit and vegetables. Fruit typically contains twice the amount of fibre as whole grains, and vegetables contain almost eight times the amount.

Be more aware of how and what you eat. Read nutrition and ingredient labels. Count your sodium intake for the day and cut out the foods that are high in salt. If an ingredient ends in -ose, it's sugar — don't eat it. Reduce your intake of processed oils. Cut out the refined and processed carbs such as white bread, sugary cereals, doughnuts, and so forth. And cut out the fast foods; they are full of excess calories because they contain high amounts of refined carbs, sodium, sugar, and processed oils.

Don't graze; eat three meals per day and enjoy them. You need to feel satisfied. Put your fork and knife down between bites and really taste the food. Pay attention to your food. Don't eat in front of the TV or computer, and don't read while you eat, because you'll be finished before you know it and you won't feel satisfied. Prepare healthy snacks, such as fruit and vegetables, for those moments when you "need something." And try to reduce your intake of chemical additives. If there is a word on the label that you can't pronounce, you probably shouldn't be eating it.

It's never too late to change. A calorie-restricted vegetarian diet improves sensitivity to insulin in comparison to a conventional diabetic diet. Furthermore, diabetics who become vegetarians experience greater loss of visceral fat and reductions in both concentrations of cytokines and oxidative stress. The addition of exercise training increases the effects of the vegetarian diet. If you must be a meat-eater, then you need to counteract the negative effects. This can be done by emphasizing the intake of antioxidants, eating less-contaminated meat, and reducing calories.

Ya Gotta Detoxify . . .

To reduce the body burden on our detoxification system, we can reduce our xenobiotic intake by eating organic foods and those lower in the food chain. Eating a balanced diet, vegetarian or vegan, Mediterranean or Paleolithic, also increases intake of foods that contain the antioxidants necessary for detoxification.

In chapter 7 we reviewed the two phases of detoxification. Phase 1 prepares the chemicals for Phase 2, which makes them water soluble so that the kidneys can excrete them. Many drugs, and even chemicals from charbroiled meats, increase Phase 1 activity, with little or no induction of Phase 2 enzymes. When Phase 1 is faster than Phase 2, toxic by-products may accumulate. Alternatively, some foods induce several Phase 2 enzyme activities, which enhance detoxification. These foods include cruciferous vegetables (broccoli, Brussels sprouts, cauliflower, cabbage) as well as garlic oil, rosemary, soy, and red grape skins. The ability of these foods to induce detoxification enzymes is retained even when cooked. Phase 2 is also enhanced by curcumin, found in turmeric.

Enhancement of Phase 2 activity helps to explain the ability of fruits and vegetables to protect against many cancers. In general, this increase in Phase 2 supports better detoxification and helps to promote and maintain a healthy balance between Phase 1 and Phase 2 activities.

Here's some more data to make you think: the logic has always been that because obesity leads to the development of so many diseases, losing weight should obviously reduce the risks. However, many observational studies have paradoxically reported that weight loss is actually associated with an *increased* risk of cardiovascular disease, dementia, and total mortality. Why would this happen? The answer is that weight loss induces the release of fat-stored chemicals such as POPs, organochlorines, and pesticides into the bloodstream. It doesn't matter whether the weight loss is from a low-calorie diet or bariatric surgery. Pollutant concentrations will increase in the blood with each 10 percent of body weight lost, and they can last up to 10 years. Adding to this risk is the fact that the POP body burden is already significantly higher in obese than in lean individuals.

The healthiest way to lose weight is with a vegetarian or vegan diet to supply nutritional support for detoxification, plus an increased intake of antioxidants to reduce the likelihood of oxidative stress. However, because POPs are resistant to natural detoxification systems, an appropriate weight-loss program should also include active detoxification efforts to facilitate reduction of the POP body burden.

Detoxification

There are many detoxification remedies with little or no scientific validation. The bottom line is that in order for a program to claim success as a detoxification method, there must be a measured reduction in levels of chemical pollutants, demonstrated by sound scientific methodology. Indeed, the literature is limited on methods to lower POP levels.

One way the body tries to get rid of chemicals that it cannot switch to a water-soluble form is to have the liver excrete them into the intestine, via bile. This is known as enterohepatic circulation. It is not very efficient, because once the chemical enters the small intestine, it is likely just to be reabsorbed. There have been some animal and human case studies of techniques that interfere with the enterohepatic circulation of some POPs. Certain drugs absorb the bile and are themselves excreted in the stool. One of these drugs is cholestyramine, an older medication used to lower cholesterol. Another drug shown to be effective is a non-absorbable dietary fat substitute called olestra. Fibre also works in the same way.

Sauna Therapy

Detoxification can be enhanced by a technique called heat depuration. Simply put, this is a technique that mobilizes chemicals from fat and enhances their excretion via sweat. The simplest way to heat the body to promote sweating is a dry sauna. There are different types of saunas, each claiming to be superior. One is the traditional Finnish type, which entails heating rocks to warm up the sauna. A more recent version uses far-infrared rays, the same rays that make us feel hot in sunlight (not to be confused with ultraviolet rays, which can cause skin cancer).

Over the years, many studies have looked at the physiologic responses of the cardiovascular system to sauna therapy. Usually the heart pumps five to 10 percent of the blood to the skin. With sauna therapy there is a dramatic increase of cardiac output to the skin, increasing it to 50 percent. The deep-body temperature increases significantly, by 1 degree Celsius. The heart rate goes up but blood pressure drops slightly. Even in patients with heart failure, cardiac output increases.

The body excretes many toxic heavy metals through sweat, such as bismuth, cadmium, mercury, chromium, thallium, and uranium. Women tend to be better at excreting them than men. Plastics come out in sweat as well. Until recently there had been just two observational studies using sweating to detoxify mercury and lead. Since the body excretes drugs in sweat, this knowledge led to the idea that patients could eliminate other unwanted xenobiotics more easily via sweat induction using the sauna. Physical exercise prior to sauna use activates fat, which releases stored xenobiotics. We now have several uncontrolled case studies demonstrating that sweating subsequent to exercise can reduce the xenobiotic load, including PCBs.

There are several different protocols for heat depuration. The common denominator is exercise followed by sauna. The prescribed length of time in the sauna varies. Daily saunas are recommended, but this raises concerns about possible dehydration and loss of essential minerals. However, none of the studies report any evidence for dehydration. Some protocols employ various supplements and replacement of minerals during therapy.

Sauna therapy also reduces oxidative stress. It is beneficial for patients with chronic widespread pain such as in fibromyalgia, rheumatoid arthritis, and ankylosing spondylitis. It improves vascular function in patients with coronary risk factors such as hypertension, high cholesterol, diabetes, and smoking, and it can even be beneficial for patients with congestive heart failure. Repeated sauna use can also help reduce levels of triglycerides and low-density lipoprotein while increasing levels of high-density lipoprotein.

Because of the heat load from saunas, patients with unstable angina, recent heart attack, decompensated heart failure, cardiac arrhythmia, uncontrolled hypertension, and severe aortic stenosis should not try sauna therapy. It is not risky for patients with hypertension, coronary heart disease, and congestive heart failure if they are medicated and in a stable condition. Some medications may exacerbate low blood pressure, which could be of concern in a sauna. If you have any of these conditions, contact your physician before starting sauna therapy.

Elimination Diets

Adverse reactions to foods is another emerging issue, frequently seen in patients with environmental sensitivities. Food intolerance is another controversial condition. It includes intolerance to gluten and appears to be initiated by antibodies called IgG, which are different from those involved in classical allergies (IgE). The controversy is partly because conventional skin-prick testing, while accurate for classical food allergies, cannot identify food intolerances.

People commonly make IgG antibodies to foods. Measuring them is a useful screening technique to identify foods for elimination. But food intolerance is only diagnosed following an elimination and rechallenge diet. The elimination diet consists of completely removing a number of foods simultaneously to see if the symptoms are reduced. After two to four weeks, reintroducing the foods back into the diet, one food at a time, helps identify which are triggering symptoms. Milk, wheat, eggs, and corn are the most common causes of food sensitivities, but developing a specific food intolerance also depends on which foods are eaten the most often.

Adverse response to foods is immunological and inflammatory. For those with food sensitivities, eating certain common foods can trigger multiple symptoms. It is associated with a wide range of inflammatory conditions, including migraine headaches, eosinophilic esophagitis, and irritable bowel syndrome. Following an elimination diet based on IgG antibody testing is an effective strategy for reducing the frequency and severity of symptoms.

Gluten Sensitivity

Celiac disease is an autoimmune small bowel disease triggered in genetically predisposed individuals by the ingestion of gluten. The exposure to gluten provokes the release of antibodies against it, with an inflammatory response in the small intestine that leads to severe pathological changes, easily identified by biopsy. Gluten is found in wheat, rye, and barley, and often in oats because of contamination. Some people have the same antibodies against gluten but do not develop the classical pathology changes. The elimination and rechallenge trial can prove gluten intolerance.

Symptoms are provoked by an immune response that affects the brain, the gastrointestinal system, and sometimes the skin. They include:

- [ ] gastrointestinal symptoms: abdominal pain, heartburn, diarrhea, constipation, and nausea
- [ ] neurological symptoms: headache, musculoskeletal pain, cognitive complaints ("brain fog"), tingling and/or numbness in hands and feet, and fatigue
- [ ] skin rash.

Diet is one of the most difficult parts of the nine-point plan to implement because it requires constant self-discipline and daily planning. It is also one of the most essential parts, because if followed properly, it should eliminate extra weight, xenobiotics, and foods that cause adverse reactions. At the same time it will provide high amounts of appropriate nutrients such as antioxidants and rebalance the microbiome. These changes will reduce oxidative stress and systemic inflammation and help promote detoxification and mitochondrial biogenesis. On the other hand, it won't be very effective without the other parts of the program — especially exercise.

CHAPTER 20

HOW TO EXERCISE

The secret of getting ahead is getting started.

— Mark Twain

Calorie restriction without malnutrition extends the lifespan in a wide range of organisms, including yeasts, worms, flies, and mammals, by lowering free radical production by the mitochondria. In mammals, including humans, calorie restriction has repeatedly been shown to retard the onset and incidence of age-related diseases. It maintains function and extends both lifespan and health, including brain and behavioural function. It does so, at least in part, by inducing mitochondrial biogenesis. Furthermore, well-nourished calorie restriction induces it even more so when in combination with exercise.

We know that exercise can help to lose weight, enhance mood, mobilize fat to aid in detoxification, improve the metabolism of lipids, increase insulin sensitivity, reduce chronic inflammation (cytokines), increase oxygen supply to the cells, and promote mitochondrial function and biogenesis. The best exercise is aerobic because it increases the oxygen supply everywhere, including the brain.

How Hard Do You Have to Exercise?

Ideally we should exercise daily, but what's the minimum amount of exercise required? There are people who claim to be physically active because they go up and down the stairs so many times during the day doing the laundry and taking care of the house, they walk to work, or they walk the dog once or twice a day. I teach my patients to take their pulse to measure their heart rate. If it goes up enough after these activities, then they are working out aerobically. But usually performing routine household activities is not hard enough or long enough exercise to be considered an aerobic workout.

Aerobic exercise demands an increase in available oxygen, resulting in an increase in the pulse and respiratory rate. The Canadian Society for Exercise Physiology has developed evidence-based guidelines for aerobic exercise. These guidelines are endorsed by the Public Health Agency of Canada and are identical to those used by both U.S. Health and Human Services and the World Health Organization. The guidelines say:

- [ ] Adults aged 18 to 64 should do at least 150 minutes (2.5 hours) of moderate-intensity aerobic physical activity per week or at least 75 minutes of vigorous aerobic physical activity per week, or an equivalent combination of the two
- [ ] The minimum duration of aerobic exercise per session should be 10 minutes
- [ ] Older adults with poor mobility should perform physical activity to enhance balance and prevent falls three or more days per week;
- [ ] Muscle-strengthening activities involving major muscle groups should be done on two or more days a week
- [ ] When older adults cannot do the recommended amounts of physical activity because of health conditions, they should be as physically active as their abilities and condition allows.

Measuring the Intensity of a Workout

What are moderate or vigorous activities? How do you measure the intensity of a physical activity? Intensity is the level of effort required by a person to do an activity. The better shape you are in, the less effort is required. Intensity of exercise is relative to how that physical activity affects your heart rate and breathing. There are actually two ways to measure exercise intensity to determine if what you are doing is aerobically adequate. They are (1) target heart rate, calculated from your maximum heart rate according to age, and (2) perceived exertion.

Target Heart Rate

There's a sweet spot for heart rate for every age. If you can get your heart pumping to that point, you will benefit aerobically. Less than that level provides little benefit, while raising it too high can be dangerous. In order to monitor yourself, you need to be able to take your own pulse. You can find it on your inner wrist, on the thumb side. If you have trouble finding it, ask a health care professional to teach you. Your pulse, or heart rate, is the number of beats per minute.

For moderate-intensity physical activity, your target heart rate should be 50 to 70 percent of your calculated maximum heart rate according to your age. Your goal is to exercise enough to achieve a heart rate of approximately 60 percent of your maximum for your age. Calculating your goal is a simple two-step process:

1. Subtract your age from 220. That's the maximum for your age.
2. Calculate 60 percent of that result. That is your target heart rate.

For vigorous-intensity physical activity, a person's target heart rate should be 70 to 85 percent of his or her maximum heart rate.

Rating Perceived Exertion

For ME/CFS patients, proceeding straight into exercise is not going to work. They need to understand where they are on a different scale. Their perception of their efforts might appear exaggerated to the rest of us, but they need to calculate their own optimal effort to be sure that they don't overexert. That would cause excessive fatigue with prolonged recovery and increased oxidative stress, making them worse.

Everyone has a different breaking point depending on the state of his or her mitochondria. Well-trained athletes can run 20 miles before they reach that point, while ME/CFS patients might last only two minutes. This is known as "hitting the wall." Once a person hits it, the mitochondria cannot maintain the energy supply any longer. The body starts breaking itself down to supply sources of fuel. This is known as the anaerobic threshold.

ME/CFS patients have impaired mitochondrial energy metabolism. They reach the anaerobic threshold within two minutes. And because they can't replace the mitochondrial energy fast enough, their exercise-capacity test scores are even worse 24 hours later. Their oxidative stress levels rise faster and stay high longer. ME/CFS patients need to pace themselves carefully, because there is more damage when they push themselves and crash. The only reliable tool these patients have to monitor and manage their exertion is their own perception. A rule of thumb for them is to exercise for two minutes, rest for five, and then repeat.

What's the Best Exercise?

What should the rest of us do for exercise? Because you want to drive more oxygen into your cells to stimulate the mitochondria, do anything that increases cardiac output. Find something that you like to do, because you need to incorporate it into your new lifestyle. Walking is a convenient and beneficial mode of exercise, whether you are physically fit or sedentary and obese. And it gets you places. Just get your heart rate up for 20 minutes every day. If there are any health concerns, you should consult with your physician first.

CHAPTER 21

THE ROLE OF SUPPLEMENTS

Let food be thy medicine and medicine be thy food.

— Hippocrates

Antioxidant Supplements

Our detoxification systems are very complex — more than a thousand antioxidants have been identified. Antioxidant supplements are "nutraceuticals," which are food products that provide beneficial heath effects. We extract them from food and package them in higher concentrations to supplement the diet. If oxidative stress is a concern for you, should you take extra antioxidants?

First we have to decide whether taking antioxidants does any good. Although antioxidant molecules counter oxidative stress in laboratory experiments, there is still some argument about whether consuming extra antioxidants actually benefits human health. Some clinical trials have found no benefit. Some researchers even argue that consuming antioxidants in excessive doses may have negative effects. But other authors have roundly criticized those trials. One of the criticisms is that only single antioxidants were used, or at best two together, rather than a cocktail of several antioxidants. The negative studies have thus taken the reductionist path of pumping a single antioxidant into a very complex system.

The best strategy to reduce oxidative stress nutritionally, even for healthy people, is to make the main course of most meals vegetables, cooked or raw. You can get your protein from nuts, legumes, grains, and seeds, or from meat. Eating lots of fruit also adds antioxidants to the diet. Consider the polluted state of the planet, your exposome (life-history exposures), your present xenobiotic load of approximately 200 chemicals, the chemical pollutants you encounter every day, and where you sit on the oxidative stress continuum. Perhaps you need to consume a larger amount of antioxidants.

What about supplements? Antioxidant supplements are not a substitute for a healthy diet and lifestyle, but given the overwhelming evidence for oxidative stress and cell damage found in acquired chronic illnesses, nobody knows whether we can obtain enough antioxidant benefits from diet alone. It would depend on our exposome, our present exposures, and how well we can detoxify. If you are thinking of taking supplements, remember that more than a thousand antioxidants have been identified. You must emphasize antioxidant sources in your diet. Which additional antioxidants you should take is presently based on logical probabilities.

Mitochondrial Cocktails

Many of the supplements offered to alleviate oxidative stress are based only upon a predicted outcome and are often given in combination, as a "mitochondrial cocktail." A mitochondrial cocktail is a combination of nutraceutical compounds intended to influence mitochondrial function by targeting several pathways at the same time. The theory is that specific combinations of nutraceutical compounds are superior to taking one supplement in isolation, because then many of the biochemical pathways involved in oxidative stress can be targeted simultaneously.

There are several studies of aging on mice in which a complex dietary supplement — a "cocktail" — was used to target oxidative stress, inflammation, mitochondrial function, insulin resistance, and cell membrane integrity. These studies demonstrated a highly significant effect, reducing physical and cognitive decline and oxidative stress. There is also some evidence to suggest that combination therapies can reduce oxidative stress and improve mitochondrial function in humans. Unfortunately, the composition and dosages vary widely according to the beliefs, expertise, and targets of the prescriber, making it hard to evaluate the results.

Although the roles of the specific ingredients and their interactions are not yet clear and the individual doses may require alteration, the results of these animal and human studies have provided significant testimony that complex dietary cocktails can powerfully reduce the biomarkers of oxidative stress. Using a cocktail of supplements fits and supports the systems medicine paradigm: there is a better chance of initiating more significant change by influencing several factors in a complex system simultaneously.

However, no well-designed studies on humans published to date have been long-term. The only other evidence for effects on humans is anecdotal, and there are no reports thus far on side effects or safety. Nevertheless, improvements have been clinically observed in patients with diverse conditions such as ME/CFS, fibromyalgia, and cardiovascular disease.

Supplements or Not?

Your decision to take supplements should consider your current exposures, your exposome, and where you think you sit on the oxidative stress continuum, as well as how you apply the precautionary principle.[9] Antioxidants occur naturally in every cell in our bodies and are also found in the vegetables and fruit that we eat. However, if we add our current exposures to our exposome, it is probable that we are lacking sufficient

---

9 The precautionary principle is an ethic that dictates that when human activities might lead to morally unacceptable harm that is uncertain but scientifically plausible, actions should be taken to avoid or diminish that harm.

antioxidants to push back against the burden of pollution that keeps using them up. One way we find evidence for oxidative stress in our cells is by discovering reduced levels of antioxidants.

There is no evidence that proves that taking additional antioxidants is unhealthy or dangerous. However, the precautionary principle tells us that taking antioxidants has to be proven to be safe before they should be taken. Sometimes we choose to take things because the benefit outweighs the risk. For example, taking low doses of Aspirin has benefits for preventing cardiovascular disease but increases the risk for gastrointestinal bleeding. Whether the benefit outweighs the risk depends on each patient's circumstances. For example, if you are prone to peptic ulcers, the risk for bleeding is increased.

At least we now know that we have choices. Because I live within a mile of a major highway that 450,000 cars traverse every day, I have decided to take supplements to push back against the chemical pollutants in my environment and slow down my journey along the oxidative stress continuum. My choice to live in a major urban centre (Toronto) has to do with both personal and professional reasons. I have examined the studies and am applying my knowledge of preventive medicine to my own lifestyle, by limiting the chemical products used in my home, eating an organic vegan diet, exercising, and taking a sauna several times a week. I believe that taking supplements will provide additional support to all my other efforts to slow down my journey on the continuum.

Whether you take these supplements or not should be decided based on which side of the precautionary principle you are on. Should you take these supplements because you probably have oxidative stress, or should you not take them because their benefit is not solidly proven and there is no evidence that there is no risk for harm? Bear in mind that every one of these nutraceuticals already exists in every cell in your body. The idea is to push back against the burden of pollution that keeps using them up.

Observations from My Practice

Over the past five to 10 years, the published literature has exploded in its attention to the damage caused by xenobiotics, inadequate detoxification, and oxidative stress. I witness the clinical results of this damage every day in my medical practice. Several years ago, N.K. came to see me because of chronic low-back pain that was gradually becoming more severe and more widespread. He was starting to experience pain in his neck, shoulders, upper back, and arms, and he had 15 of the 18 positive tender points found in fibromyalgia. N.K. was otherwise in good health. He was a 60-year-old who exercised regularly, followed an organic vegan diet, and was not overweight. His previous health history was normal except for a severe allergy to peanuts. His environmental exposure history was not unusual, and scented products had been eliminated in his home and workplace. N.K. was frustrated and worried about the progression of his pain, but he was reluctant to take the medications usually recommended to manage chronic widespread pain.

N.K. was also educated about public health. We discussed systems biology and oxidative stress, and he became keenly interested in trying an antioxidant cocktail. The results of that trial of treatment were remarkable. Within weeks his widespread pain had diminished significantly. Since then, the cocktail has been tried by many other patients. Positive results are often observed, but usually only after several months. While it can be beneficial, there is no doubt that taking antioxidant supplements is only one part of a larger therapeutic program. N.K.'s lifestyle already included most of the nine-step program, but he needed that nutraceutical boost. The systems medicine approach is multifactorial.

The cocktail prescribed to my patients when they are also following the nine-point program includes the following:

- [ ] CoQ10 (150–300 mg)
- [ ] alpha-lipoic acid (600 mg)
- [ ] L-carnitine or acetyl-L-carnitine (500–3,000 mg)

- ☐ magnesium (400–800 mg)
- ☐ N-acetyl-cysteine (500 mg).

When we want to promote mitochondrial biogenesis, we suggest adding:

- ☐ resveratrol (40 mg one to three times daily)
- ☐ quercitin (100 mg one to three times daily).

We also frequently add:

- ☐ melatonin (3–9 mg)
- ☐ fish oils (omega-3 fatty acids)
- ☐ curcumin/turmeric (1,200 mg), for its anti-inflammatory effect
- ☐ creatine, to enhance energy production.

Nutraceutical recommendations are somewhat empirical and must be individualized. If you try adding supplements, they should be introduced in a stepwise fashion and increased slowly to identify and minimize potential intolerances. Treatment should be supervised by a knowledgeable health care professional.

Studies confirm that the more multifaceted the program, the more beneficial the effect. In my experience, I get the best results when the patients buy in and follow the treatment program concepts inspired by my grandmother: environmental control with reduced pollutant exposures, detoxification, clean diet, aerobic exercise followed by sauna, calorie restriction to reduce BMI (if appropriate), nutritional support provided by a nutrient-dense diet, and whatever supplements each patient might require, including the various ingredients of a mitochondrial cocktail.

CHAPTER 22

PATIENT STORIES

Stories are meant to comfort the afflicted and afflict the comfortable.
— Finley Peter Dunne

When P.D. first came to see me, he was a 40-year-old man with a 10-year history of chronic fatigue that became so bad with exertion that recovery took more than 24 hours. He had chronic widespread pain in his muscles and joints, frequent headaches, heartburn, mood swings, and cognitive complaints: decreased attention span, poor concentration, poor short-term memory, difficulty finding words, and distractibility. His sleep was disturbed; it took him up to an hour to fall asleep, he woke up frequently, and he did not feel well rested in the morning. He was sensitive to heat, cold, noise, bright lights, stress, and multiple chemical scents. He had a long-standing history of allergies to dust mites and shellfish.

P.D.'s environmental exposure history revealed that he had been a pilot for five years before working in an office building, which he described as having poor air quality, even according to his colleagues. Symptoms of headache, sore throat, nasal congestion, and cough flared up at work and reduced when he left the building. There was a no-scent policy, but it was not strictly enforced or respected by some colleagues. Both work environments demonstrated significant indoor air pollutant exposures that likely pushed him along the oxidative stress continuum.

His main complaints affecting his quality of life were the fatigue and the pain. Previous doctors had diagnosed chronic fatigue syndrome (ME/CFS), fibromyalgia, multiple chemical sensitivities (MCS), and gastroesophageal reflux disease (GERD). On physical examination I found generalized tenderness. He was not overweight. We assessed his fatigue and pain, using validated questionnaires, and found evidence for reduced function and disability. P.D. was still able to work full-time as an administrator. He also managed to play hockey once a week, with subsequent increased fatigue and pain for 48 hours following the activity. But his overall quality of life was otherwise markedly reduced. Prior to the onset of illness he had no health complaints and was very physically active. P.D. had the pattern, including multi-morbidity, which provided evidence for significant oxidative stress and reduced number and function of mitochondria.

Because he had MCS, P.D. was already trying to avoid obvious airborne chemical exposures. I placed him on a treatment program of aerobic exercise for 20 minutes daily followed by a sauna, a vegan organic diet, and a "mitochondrial cocktail" of supplements. The result was a slow but gradual clinical improvement. Within six months P.D. stated, "I feel normal again." His only remaining complaints were mild classical allergy symptoms of nasal congestion in the winter, associated with dust mite exposure and dry air.

Not all patients do as well as P.D. Some don't respond to the treatment and others refuse or are unable to buy in to the lifestyle changes required. But in my experience the program helps many patients, at least somewhat.

B.C. is a middle-aged woman with long-standing ME/CFS. Here's how she described her experience after six months of treatment:

> Whether I feel like it or not, I go to the pool three times a week, get into the water and swim and the water is always so soft. The day I swim and the following day as well, my level of exhaustion is less and my level of pain is less also. And overall,

I am exhausted less frequently. When I am, I no longer feel shattered — instead I just feel tired. Normal tired.

At times I remember what it is to feel normal. From that feeling, I can understand better why I do not function well. At my very best moments, I can feel all the systems in the body waking up. When I eat, my body says "Thank you!" as the nutrients are somehow able to be received, absorbed, and used by the cells.

When I walk to the pool from the parking lot, my limbs no longer feel weighted down with cement. I have the energy after swimming to wash my hair. I can stand in the shower and the drops of water do not hurt my skin. I can stand and talk to a neighbour without looking for a chair. I can go up the stairs without lactic acid filling my legs.

I feel good when walking down the street. I want to see the people. I have the energy to be alive. I want to engage in life. I love to just feel normal.

Everything in the world is still too loud, too fast, too bright, too harsh, too unforgiving. I get a bit disoriented. Memory is still a problem. The swimming routine cannot be discontinued even for a few days. Otherwise, I have to start over again from square one.

B.C. and P.D. are two example cases of response to the common sense systems approach to therapy for chronic illness. B.C. is still not healthy but is appreciative of the improvement in her quality of life. We do not yet have all the answers we need for successful treatment for most chronic conditions. Presently our treatments are rudimentary, but by changing to a systems medicine approach, we are making improvements in people's lives that the standard model cannot achieve. By changing paradigms, we are now starting to look for and find answers in the right places.

If You Don't Change Your Lifestyle, Your Life Won't Change

F.T. was an extremely obese woman who complained of chronic fatigue and pain. Her medical history, already described in chapter 17, was complex, complicated, and typical. She had chronic multiple symptoms from multiple systems. She was obese, diabetic, hypertensive, and asthmatic, and she had frequent respiratory infections. She was also depressed, frustrated, and bitter.

> The worst doctors already think they know what is wrong with you. They either dismiss your concerns or symptoms that don't fit their theory, or they don't ask questions, or they tell you nothing is wrong. I have had so many doctors treat me like I am stupid. It shuts me down. I feel intimidated. I feel angry and I resent going to them only to feel frustrated. I also hate it when they say something mean. I feel defenceless and, in one case, I was called fat six times during the consultation.

The challenge was to get F.T. to stop feeling like a victim of the medical system, to take control of her life and to change it. Empowering patients requires imparting knowledge. Therefore, the first step in F.T.'s chronic care management was to educate her, to enable her to make informed choices on her own, without the influence of her emotions, in order to make the changes required to manage her chronic illness better.

F.T. had very low self-esteem. Although that could easily be explained by the childhood bullying and abuse, she also weighed almost 300 pounds. She told me, "Even my own husband is repulsed by me!" Is it any wonder that many psychiatrists had failed to improve her self-esteem? They don't treat obesity, fatigue, or chronic pain. Was F.T. mentally ill to think that she was repulsive to her husband and ridiculed by society? What about the effect of all her cytokines on her brain function? Maybe her pain and obesity were also influenced by pollution and oxidative stress. And maybe she needed more mitochondria.

What is required to treat chronic illness is a systems medicine approach. F.T. was offered a series of long appointments, with the goal being that she would develop the tools to make herself feel physically and mentally better. She bought in because she was taught the concepts in this book and chose to follow the nine-point program. Her visits with me were patient-centred. Teaching F.T. required more than imparting the latest medical knowledge. I also had to understand her illness experience in order to help her deal with obstacles to change when they occurred. Chronic illness is a biopsychosocial, multisystem, chemical, organelle, cellular, and organ pathological process.

F.T. and I became partners: her care was not just patient-focused; it became person-focused too. She received emotional support, praise for her achievements, and problem-solving guidance for her failures. Most of all, she became educated and motivated to change. She developed confidence and trust, which eventually led to her feeling enabled. As a result, she made informed choices and followed through. And I cheered and applauded her achievements along the way.

F.T. began to walk every day, monitoring her effort by taking her own pulse. She became a vegan and bought only organic food. She cleaned her home environment to reduce the chemical exposures. She enhanced the detoxification process by taking frequent saunas, and she encouraged cell repair by taking a handful of prescribed antioxidant supplements twice a day.

She asked questions and maintained a journal of her experiences. I never passed judgment on her occasional lapses in self-discipline, and eventually she stopped doing that too. But what helped most to keep F.T. motivated to maintain the self-discipline of lifestyle change was the physical rewards. Her pain was markedly reduced, her energy increased, and she began to lose weight steadily. Her IBS and GERD symptoms disappeared. She now sleeps better, her mind is clearer, and her mood is more stable. She went through an entire winter without having any episodes of bronchitis or pneumonia. She is less chemically sensitive. Her medications have been reduced or discontinued. And she no longer feels repulsive to her husband.

I know what to do. I want to do it and I believe in the treatment prescribed as a formula to overall better health. When I follow it, I am virtually pain-free, happy, clear-headed, my diabetes is well managed, my digestive system works well and I lose weight.

F.T. has maintained the program for more than one year.

So, is it physical or mental?

PART VI

THE ENVIRONMENT OF MEDICINE

NAME⎽⎽⎽⎽⎽⎽⎽⎽⎽⎽⎽⎽⎽⎽⎽⎽⎽⎽⎽⎽⎽⎽⎽⎽ AGE⎽⎽⎽⎽⎽⎽⎽
ADDRESS⎽⎽⎽⎽⎽⎽⎽⎽⎽⎽⎽⎽⎽⎽⎽⎽⎽⎽⎽⎽ DATE⎽⎽⎽⎽⎽⎽

☐ LABEL
REFILL 0 1 2 3 4 5   ⎽⎽⎽⎽⎽⎽⎽⎽⎽⎽⎽⎽⎽⎽⎽⎽⎽⎽
                                      (SIGNATURE)

CHAPTER 23

THE POLITICS OF MEDICINE

When we least expect it, life sets us a challenge to test our courage and willingness to change.

— Paulo Coelho, *The Devil and Miss Prym*

Writing this book enabled me to synthesize my experiences as an environmental physician, and I am awestruck by what I have seen. Looking back, I can thank some of my colleagues for their skepticism and their negative behaviours because they challenged me to spend countless hours in the medical library searching the literature, which is now only a few clicks away on my computer. I have worked on this book every day for more than two years, but increasingly it feels as if I have been surfing on the crest of a giant wave of new and fascinating (yet frightening) information and changing paradigms. The biopsychosocial environment has evolved, the genotype of our children and adult health patterns are changing, and the practice of medicine will have to change accordingly.

Multiple exposures have considerable impacts on unborn children that partially depend on how well they can detoxify. Given this reality, how can toxicologists still stick to the old paradigm? Multiple exposures contribute to oxidative stress and the likelihood of developing a chronic medical condition. How can the reductionists deny the impact on multiple systems and the concepts of systems medicine? And how do we keep up with the tidal wave of new data?

People have divergent opinions and they tend to argue with those whose opinions differ from their own. In the courtroom it's not about who's right, it's about who wins. And politicians are no different. Why were complaints published in prestigious science journals such as *Nature* that climate scientists at Environment Canada were forbidden from sharing their work at conferences and talking about published research? If you believe that interpretation of scientific data is not subject to political influence when being considered for public policy, consider this: according to an October 2009 survey, 75 percent of Democrats in the United States see solid evidence that the average temperature on Earth has been getting warmer over the past few decades, compared to just 37 percent of Republicans. Why should political affiliation make a difference to the acceptance of science?

Recently while sitting on the patio of my condo, I noticed a man spraying the grass in the nearby common area with a brown liquid. When I asked, he informed me that he was spraying the weeds with an iron-containing compound permitted by the City of Toronto, even though Toronto had banned the cosmetic use of herbicides. I jokingly asked if he was actually killing the weeds or just putting them to sleep. He replied in a frustrated manner that it didn't work as well as the banned herbicides and that it was 10 times more expensive. When I answered that at least it wasn't killing people, he responded that the banned herbicides didn't either. When I told him that I practised environmental medicine and that the science said they should be banned, he became angry and told me I was wrong.

I walked back into my home, not bothering to explain to him that the literature shows a relationship between herbicides and some cancers, neurodegenerative disorders, and oxidative stress. Likely, his employers had reassured him that it was perfectly safe for him to apply the banned herbicides, and that the evidence supporting the adverse health effects was just junk science.

Meanwhile, the experiment in human chemical evolution continues, and no one has signed the consent form. There are 23,000 chemicals in Canada on the Domestic Substance List, chemicals in use for more than 20 years yet never evaluated for toxicity. Under the federal Chemicals Management Plan (CMP), which began in 2006, categorization identified 200 chemical substances that are potentially harmful to human health or the environment. These chemicals represent the highest priorities for risk assessment and appropriate controls. According to the CMP website, the Government of Canada will use existing tools and regulations to challenge industry to provide new information about how it is managing these 200 chemical substances.

The government went so far as to form a CMP Stakeholder Advisory Council, a multi-stakeholder committee, to contribute to implementation of that process. Its members represent Aboriginal groups, consumer groups, environment NGOs (non-government organizations), health NGOs, industry (including associations, producers, and users), and labour. None of the members of this council has any medical training. They know the Environmental Health Committee of the College of Family Physicians exists. Shouldn't people who might get sick from the environment be represented too? Aren't they stakeholders? Why isn't the college on this advisory council?

Given the evidence for low-dose exposures and epigenetic changes, we all need to ask what standards the government applies to assess for potential harm. More important, multiple exposures to low levels of pollutants, in particular in unborn or newborn children, have never been tested for safety, and we need to figure out how even to carry out such an assessment with any scientific accuracy. Our present methodology focuses on testing single exposures, which clearly does not accurately reflect real-world exposures.

In December 1999 the European Commission adopted a strategy on assessing endocrine disruptors. Eight years later it produced its third progress report, which stated that it had screened and evaluated 575 chemicals for their endocrine-disrupting effects. The European Commission established a preliminary priority list. Out of the 575 substances, 320 substances showed evidence or potential evidence for endocrine-disrupting effects, 118 are high-production-volume or highly persistent substances with evidence or potential evidence of endocrine-disrupting effects, and 109 of them are already regulated or under review in existing legislation. Sounds like our European neighbours are well looked after — except for the fact that there are no scientific studies that determine safe levels of environmental exposure, or the maximum allowable body burden, when the real world of multiple exposures and additive and synergistic effects is considered. The European Commission's website specifically states: "In the coming years, further legislative work may be done on endocrine disruptors."

In 1996 the U.S. Congress legislated that the Environmental Protection Agency (EPA) initiate the Endocrine Disruptor Screening Program, to screen pesticide chemicals and environmental contaminants for their potential to affect the endocrine systems of humans and wild-life. In 2009 the EPA announced that it had finalized its Tier 1 battery of analyses. Now that screening is underway, in Tier 2 the EPA is preparing to review responses, make decisions, and request additional testing as needed. Tier 2 will involve multiple stakeholders to determine whether further testing is required to find specific doses that are toxic, for regulatory actions. Further testing? How are they ever going to determine those doses when several hundred varying chemical exposures are occurring at the same time?

In June 2009 the Endocrine Society, comprising 14,000 hormone researchers and medical specialists in more than a hundred countries, warned: "Even infinitesimally low levels of exposure to endocrine-disrupting chemicals — indeed, any level of exposure at all — may cause endocrine or reproductive abnormalities, particularly if exposure occurs during a critical developmental window. Low doses may even exert more potent effects than higher doses." In November 2009 the American Medical Association's House of Delegates approved a resolution that called on the federal government to minimize the public's exposure to BPA and other endocrine-disrupting chemicals. This resolution was originally put forward by the Endocrine Society, the American Society for

Reproductive Medicine, and the American College of Obstetricians and Gynecologists.

Two years later, eight medical societies representing approximately 40,000 research scientists and clinicians in the fields of reproductive biology, endocrinology, reproductive medicine, genetics, and developmental biology sent an open letter to the Food and Drug Administration and the EPA. They offered the expertise of their societies to serve on panels to assess the risk of specific chemicals through evaluation of the data and to develop new testing guidelines and protocols, because "currently accepted testing paradigms and government review practices are inadequate for chemicals with hormone-like actions." These societies included:

- ☐ American Society of Human Genetics
- ☐ American Society for Reproductive Medicine
- ☐ Endocrine Society
- ☐ Genetics Society of America
- ☐ Society for Developmental Biology
- ☐ Society for Pediatric Urology
- ☐ Society for the Study of Reproduction
- ☐ Society for Gynecological Investigation.

How much longer is all this going to take? Needless to say, the chemical industry is also a major stakeholder. A 2006 review of 130 in vivo studies regarding the endocrine disrupting effects of BPA in the scientific literature found the following:

- ☐ Over 90 percent of the 109 government-funded in vivo studies conclude that there are observable effects in response to low doses of BPA
- ☐ Most of the studies that reported an absence of adverse effects had used one particular type of rat as the test animal. Known as the CD-SD rat, it is relatively unresponsive to estrogens except at high doses. No study using the CD-SD rat reported finding any

effect that would be detected in a standard toxicological study
conducted for risk-assessment purposes
- ☐ Of the 21 studies that reported negative findings, 11 were funded by industry
- ☐ No studies reporting positive findings were funded by industry.

The results of science studies are supposed to be unbiased, yet clearly they can be influenced by how they are designed and who funded them. This same review also concluded that the weight of evidence based on published studies concerning low-dose effects of BPA in experimental animals demonstrates the need for reevaluation of the acceptable level of daily human exposure in the United States, which is 50 micrograms per kilogram per day (mcg/kg/day). Canada's provisional tolerable daily intake (TDI) is 25 mcg/kg.

So what is the acceptable TDI for a pregnant woman? Since BPA crosses the placenta, what is the acceptable level for an unborn child? What about the additive or synergistic effects from all the other exposures in the real world? How long should we wait for the various government agencies to decide? Do you think it's possible that they could be influenced in their decision-making by the chemical industry? How would our society ever cope without all the conveniences of our chemical world?

To its credit, in 2008 Canada began the Canadian Healthy Infant Longitudinal Development (CHILD) Study, which enrolled 5,000 children, starting prenatally, and followed them for five years. The hypothesis is that exposure to indoor pollutants, including both chemical and microbiological agents, interact with host genetic, hormonal, metabolic, psychosocial, physiological, nutritional, and immunological factors, which increases the risk of allergy and asthma in infancy and early childhood. While this study is to be commended, it clearly does not encompass the other long-term health concerns reviewed above. And the duration should be extended. Why stop after five years? What about those exposures and possible effects in puberty, adolescence, and young adulthood?

Public health decisions should be based on studies that use appropriate protocols. We need to develop new protocols, but how do we test the effects of hundreds of chemicals at levels that fluctuate individually yet are constantly mixing together?

The chemical industry clearly has economic interests and the right and obligation to be involved in the evaluation and decision-making process. It has a financial and moral responsibility as well. Despite the industry's denials, chemical pollution is making people ill and making a mess of our planet. But we all buy and use their chemical products.

How can we end our exposures to plastics, fire retardants, solvents, and stain repellents? How can we stop burning fossil fuels? Who is responsible for cleaning up this mess? Right-wing politicians deny that there is a problem so that they are not faced with increasing government influence on private enterprise. And left-wing policies can't afford to stifle industry — the lifeline of industry is economic and driven by consumer demand.

What Have We Learned from the Sumerians?

The end of the human race will be that it will eventually die of civilization.
— Ralph Waldo Emerson

Our hunter-gatherer ancestors roamed the Fertile Crescent, a horseshoe-shaped area that extended from the Persian Gulf up to the Euphrates and Tigris Rivers in present-day Iraq, and back down to Israel and Egypt. The climate was temperate, and continuously flooding rivers made the fertile soil ideal for early revolutions in agriculture and farming. For reasons that we can only theorize, there was a transition in human behaviour from foraging to planting gardens for food. About 8,000 years ago our gardens evolved to become a major source of food, the nomadic way of life gave way to farming cultures, and there was a transition to permanent settlement and community living.

The Sumerians formed one of the earliest urban societies to emerge successfully as a dominant culture, more than 5,000 years ago. They grew wheat and barley and dug ditches from rivers to irrigate their crops. As the population grew, they developed city communities, and some people were no longer farmers. Instead there were those who became weavers, worked metal or leather, or built the roads and canals. In order to organize themselves, they developed a government, including a monarchy and a bureaucracy. They learned to keep written records and to do mathematics, and they developed a calendar to be efficient in their record-keeping. Present-day archaeological sites of the ancient Sumerian cities still provide testimony to their great civilization.

To support this new type of society, each farmer was required to grow much more produce than he needed personally, because he now had to supply food for those who no longer farmed for a living. However, there was a problem with salinization of the land used for farming. When the water brought in by the canal system evaporated, it left behind layers of salt. Repeated flooding over time brought even more salt to the soil, so that eventually the wheat crops could no longer grow well. The farmers switched from wheat to barley, but eventually even those crops diminished as the soil became increasingly unfit for food production. It was enough to cause hunger, malnutrition, and disease. There was major depopulation, leading to the collapse of Sumerian culture. No longer capable of defending themselves, they were swallowed up by invaders.

The solution to the problem would have been to farm somewhere else. Why didn't they? It was obvious to the Sumerians that the land was changing: their written records describe the earth turning white, and they did change their crop. The obvious solution would have required financial and social changes in order to alter the infrastructure of roads and canals and relocate farms. It would have taken years and required unbiased foresight and sacrifice. The Sumerians needed to change the status quo, but as a society, they chose not to. As a result, one of the first significant civilizations in our brief history perished, at least in part because of self-poisoning of their environment and subsequent refusal to alter their lifestyle.

Inconvenient Change

We could have saved the Earth but we were too damned cheap.
— Kurt Vonnegut

The Sumerians were an intelligent, hard-working, dynamic, and progressive people. What is remarkable about this historical event is that it provides the first evidence of significant, long-lasting, destructive environmental impact from human activities. It also provides the first evidence for human resistance to inconvenient change, and our tendency for bureaucratic decision making to be shortsighted, driven by politics and economics, and ultimately destructive to the society at large.

Unfortunately, some things about humans have yet to evolve. Our problem is not over-farming and salinization; instead we over-consume, and our chemicals are more numerous than salt, and more complex. There are more of us making a larger mess, so that now we have contaminated our planet to the point that we have changed the weather systems, the air we breathe, the food we eat, and our water supply. We even contaminate our unborn children and have altered the behaviour of our gene pool. Nevertheless, as individuals, we refuse to change. Our bureaucrats, politicians, and stakeholders also continue to be shortsighted, driven by politics and economics, and ultimately destructive to our society. As stated metaphorically so well by David Suzuki, "We're in a giant car heading towards a brick wall and everyone is arguing over where they're going to sit."

Consumerians

We learn from history that we do not learn from history.
— Georg Wilhelm Friedrich Hegel

Although the planet Earth has been spinning and revolving around the sun for billions of years, modern man has existed for only the past

10,000 years. The Sumerian civilization self-destructed and is extinct, but Earth continues its relentless revolutions around the sun. What have we learned? History teaches us that, while Earth will continue to spin around the sun, one day our civilization will no longer dominate or even be present on this planet. It may be sooner than we think, because we are heading down the same path to self-destruction as the Sumerians. Future archaeologists and historians may perhaps refer to our no-longer-existing civilization as "the Consumerians."

Given that we can't depend on our government, industry, or fellow consumers to change, where can you go for help to slow down, stop, or even reverse your trip along the oxidative stress continuum? How will you protect your children, including those not yet conceived?

The Battle Continues . . .

In 2011 I saw a new patient, L.E., a happily married woman with two children in her mid-forties, because of a three-year history of multiple physical and mental complaints. Prior to the onset of her illness, she had led a healthy lifestyle, was a vegetarian, exercised regularly, and practised tai chi. Her medical and psychosocial history was uneventful. Before the onset of her illness, she had begun to observe some nasal and chest congestion in certain areas of her workplace, which she then avoided. One of those locations was another building that she visited occasionally in order to work on certain projects. She was transferred to that building three years later and her symptoms increased. When at work, she began to experience headaches, difficulty concentrating, a burning sensation in her eyes and chest, and greater difficulty breathing. There were complaints about the air quality from other employees as well.

L.E. then began to notice that her symptoms could be provoked in other locations, mainly from exposure to scented products. She was working in an office environment without a scent-free policy. The office was connected to a factory on the same floor that manufactured heavy machinery. Her employers provided her temporary accommodation by allowing her to work from home or in a different building, but they also asked her to provide a medical opinion for support.

A physician diagnosed L.E. with sick building syndrome and environmental sensitivities. He sent a letter to her employers advising avoidance of provocative environments, in particular the building in which she had become worse. Unfortunately, the employers refused to accept these recommendations and obtained their own medical assessment from an occupational health physician. It was the latter's opinion that L.E. was not suffering from an organic illness; that it was psychogenic, likely from anxiety or phobia. He recommended that she be treated for panic disorder and phobia. It was his opinion that there was nothing physically wrong with her and that there was no risk in returning to the building in question, without any restrictions.

L.E. complied and started a return-to-work program but noted that her symptoms at work were increasing. Along with runny nose, nasal congestion, sore throat, cough, and headaches, she experienced fatigue, poor concentration, poor memory, and mental dullness. As a result a psychiatric assessment was ordered.

Amazingly, the primary diagnosis was anxiety disorder despite the fact that there were no unusual psychosocial factors past or present. Because she could lose her job, L.E. was forced to agree to return to work, which she did until she became too ill to continue. When I assessed her ability to function, she demonstrated significant disability. She had chronic fatigue, widespread pain, sleep disturbance, and poor cognition; she now felt anxious and depressed, which she attributed to being sick and disabled and having no income. She also had heartburn and symptoms of irritable bowel syndrome. She was sensitive to odours, including auto exhaust, new carpets, dry cleaning, gasoline products, perfumes, detergents, soaps, deodorizers, fabric softeners, and chlorinated swimming pools. She also described some food intolerances.

What Happened to L.E.?

L.E.'s history starts with mild symptoms provoked by exposure to certain environments. She was becoming a canary. Her physician supported a physical diagnosis (the good news), but the employer did not and obtained an unsubstantiated and misinformed psychiatric diagnosis (the bad news), thereby forcing the canary to stay in the coalmine. L.E. was showing signs of oxidative stress, limbic system hypervigilance, and sensitization of her TRPV1 receptors. The appropriate treatment should have been to avoid the biological stressors — to get out of the coalmine. Instead, the health care providers chosen by her employer likely pushed L.E. farther along the oxidative stress continuum, causing more damage that might be irreversible. She now had fibromyalgia, ME/CFS, IBS, and reflux to go along with her MCS.

I tell this story for two reasons. The first is to demonstrate that the farther we travel along the oxidative stress continuum, the more likely we are to develop multi-morbidity, poorer quality of life, and a greater dependency on the health care system. The second reason is to demonstrate that some doctors still use psychiatric illness to explain environmental sensitivities. The Cartesian reductionist paradigm states that if it's not physical, it's mental.

In 2007 I collaborated on a paper commissioned by the Canadian Human Rights Commission (CHRC), titled "The Medical Perspective on Environmental Sensitivities." Six weeks later, as a result of this paper, the CHRC designated this medical condition a disability, stating that people living with environmental sensitivities are entitled to protection under the Canadian Human Rights Act, which prohibits discrimination on the basis of disability. The CHRC encourages employers and service providers to proactively address issues of accommodation by ensuring that their workplaces and facilities are accessible for disabled persons. Included in their policy on environmental sensitivities is the following:

Successful accommodation for persons with environmental sensitivities requires innovative strategies to minimize or eliminate exposure to triggers in the environment. These may include: developing and enforcing fragrance free and chemical avoidance policies, undertaking educational programs to increase voluntary compliance with such policies, minimizing chemical use and purchasing less toxic products, and notifying employees and clients in advance of construction, re-modeling and cleaning activities. Such measures can prevent injuries and illnesses, and reduce costs and health and safety risks.

Partly as a result of this landmark decision, fragrance-free policies in the workplace and public establishments, such as hospitals and places of worship, are now becoming increasingly common, and implementation is being encouraged by organizations such as the Canadian Centre for Occupational Health and Safety and the Canadian Lung Association. The U.S. Centers for Disease Control and the Agency for Toxic Substances and Disease Registry have a scent-free policy in their own buildings, which states in part: "It is important that personnel be aware that the use of some personal care products may have detrimental effects on the health of chemically sensitive co-workers."

These social and behavioural changes have been mandated on the basis of science and law. So why did the Canadian Medical Association Journal publish an article in 2011 titled "Scent-Free Policies Generally Unjustified"? Is this just a good example of healthy debate based on conflicting science? Or is it irresponsible journalism because, taking its cue from the title, the article may give support to those who resist the initiation of or compliance with scent-free policies in public places and the workplace? This article has significant potential to cause harm. What is alarming is that the author reaches her conclusions without one single citation from the medical literature. Given the title and potentially harmful outcome, one would expect more supportive evidence than a general description of a placebo response, obtained in an interview with a psychologist from the Monell Chemical Senses Center. Is it just a coincidence that this institute — which describes itself as the world's only independent, non-profit scientific institute dedicated to interdisciplinary basic research on the senses of taste and smell — obtains funding from the tobacco and chemical fragrance industries? Why is this still happening?

The Theory of Diffusion of Innovations

In 1962 Everett Rogers described the theory of diffusion of innovations. According to this theory, a new idea, device, or method will go through a process of diffusion into the population over time. We see it in the business world, for example, in the fashion industry when there is a change in men's suit lapels or women's hairstyles. This process proceeds in phases as consumers adopt the product. It starts with the innovators. Early adopters then take on the idea or concept before the majority do, and the last group, which may never conform, are called laggards. The term *dinosaurs* is also used to describe those most resistant to change. This is seen in every aspect of business and institutional structure everywhere. There's no getting away from it. Laggards ignore or actively interfere with the transfer of knowledge, and will continue to do so forever.

Thomas Kuhn, who introduced the idea of paradigms into the public consciousness in 1962, recognized that science, instead of being neutral in its quest for truth, actually proceeds by continuously seeking confirmation of the prevailing paradigm. Unfortunately, as environmental medicine was evolving, an entrenched bias emerged. One reason for this was the attraction of alternative health care practitioners to environmental medicine. Some of these practitioners were just as locked into their own new box, rejecting the existing paradigms of conventional medicine. They tried various techniques, some of which remain unproven or unscientific, in an attempt to diagnose and treat patients with poorly understood illnesses. It was easy, then, to lump all the environmental practitioners together and "shoot all the messengers" in order to ensure that the prevalent reduction-ist and toxicology paradigms remained entrenched. To maintain those par-adigms, patients with ME/CFS, fibromyalgia, and especially MCS were mistreated.

In support of the traditional toxicology approach is the argument that, in the lab, we have been unable to consistently demonstrate sensi-tivity to chemicals. The ideal way to do so is to challenge patients with chemical exposures, using real chemicals or placebos. The best method-ology is called double-blind, meaning that neither the patients nor the observers know if the exposure is real or placebo — this should elimi-nate bias. However, the only way to mask the chemical is to either dilute it so there is no detectable odour or to mask it with another chemical. Either way, it doesn't work. Patients being studied will not react to a chemical if the level is too low. Nor can they tell the difference when the chemicals being studied and the inert placebos are both masked by a separate, possibly offending chemical.

A published review of the challenge studies concluded that MCS cannot exist. This paper appears to be objective and credible because it is titled "A Systematic Review of Provocation Studies." Systematic re-views identify, select, assess, and synthesize the findings of similar but separate studies. A systematic review is supposed to be objective. Why weren't the published studies including capsaicin-inhalation challenges in this systematic review of MCS? Those studies were published before the review and certainly appear on my computer screen when I use the same search terms. The omitted challenge studies demonstrate that MCS patients have sensitized TRPV1 receptors. Is it possible that it was thought best to ignore those studies because the results don't fit in the traditional paradigm box? Also, why didn't the authors conclude that chemical-inhalation challenge studies could not be blinded or masked properly?

What Is Wrong with These People?

An increasing number of people are sensitive to chemical pollutants but are still having a hard time getting their condition accepted by physicians because there are no clinical biological markers. These physicians continue to cling to the argument that sensitization contradicts the traditional toxicology paradigm, as if it were still a legitimate argument.

The canaries have been warning us to look at sensory receptors in the central nervous system, while the allergists denied their legitimacy simply because it did not conform to the traditional model of immune-system sensitization. The allergists and traditional toxicologists unfairly labelled these people with psychiatric illness, because they were locked into a reductionist paradigm. Hiding from criticism behind the walls of their proverbial box, these doctors refused to communicate respectfully with physicians who saw things differently, only because they were listening to, observing, and trying to help these patients.

The opinion of traditional allergists comes from a 1997 position paper on MCS of the American Academy of Allergy, Asthma and Immunology (AAAAI). The cited literature to support their position is now more than 15 years old, and it was highly selective, intended to summarize only some of the literature from an era when much of the current knowledge about MCS had not yet evolved. Note that a position paper is not the same as a literature review. It is a report that explains or justifies a point of view. None of the criteria required for an objective literature review were used in the AAAAI position paper. While the AAAAI states that its position statements are not to be considered to reflect current standards or policies after five years from date of publication, it is still available for viewing on the organization's website. More important, it is clearly out of date.

Unfortunately, this and other outdated position papers are still cited by those who continue to deny the existence of chemical sensitivities. This has frequently been my experience when I have reviewed the evidence postulated by others in order to provide an independent medical legal opinion. The impressive list of established, credible medical bodies that deny the existence of MCS can sway the opinion of judges, who are incapable of understanding the relative lack of value of outdated medical evidence and must rely on the testimony of so-called experts, while lawyers try to strengthen or diminish the weight of these opinions to influence judgments in court. The strength of the negative argument appears to be "who says" rather than what the up-to-date published evidence actually demonstrates. These position papers are old, hopelessly out-of-date, and they fail to acknowledge the evidence in this book. And they are still being cited by the laggards.

CHAPTER 24

PARADIGMS LOST

We do not see things as they are. We see them as we are.

— Anaïs Nin, *Seduction of the Minotaur*

The Vegetarian Paradigm

There has been a significant accumulation of knowledge regarding vegetarian diets and nutrition since they first entered the medical literature
in the 1960s.[10] The initial response was to question whether a vegan diet
provided sufficient nutrients and energy for human growth and reproduction. Whether it could promote optimal health was not considered.
Journals such as the *Lancet* published critical articles based in part on
conventional disdain for the alternative lifestyle practised by the hippie
protagonists of vegetarianism. At that time, the prevailing nutritional
paradigm was the study and prevention of nutritional deficiencies, but
the biased lens of the experts of that era whose knowledge was being
challenged is apparent from the titles of their publications, such as "Death
after Vegan Diet" and "Vegetarianism and Drug Users." To prevent the

---

10 Vegetarianism is here defined as a diet that excludes red meat and poultry. The many
forms of vegetarian diet range from pescetarian (includes fish but no meat) to ovo-lacto
vegetarian (includes eggs and dairy products but no animal proteins) to vegan (no animal
products at all, including honey).

expected malnutrition, the advice back then was to add considerable amounts of animal products such as eggs, milk, and dairy, which would essentially make the diet non-vegetarian. They had a point, albeit a small one. There is a risk of developing iron, calcium, or B_{12} deficiency on a completely vegetarian diet, or a protein deficiency, if it isn't executed properly.

Articles on the preventive and therapeutic aspects of vegetarian diets are now being published with greater frequency. They demonstrate modification of risk factors, reduced incidence of chronic diseases, and better management of some medical conditions such as obesity and diabetes. What happened? The paradigm of nutrition has changed from the old one of preventing nutritional deficiencies to the modern one of reducing excess intake of poor food choices. There is more emphasis on nutrient-dense, calorie-sparse diets, accenting the intake of antioxidants, fibre, and other anti-cancer nutrients that are found mainly in fruits, vegetables, and other plant-based foods. The change occurred because health patterns have changed. The world's population is increasingly overweight and becoming toxic. At the same time, our knowledge base has evolved and grown as well.

Now there are millions of vegetarians in all walks of life. People are more knowledgeable. Labels containing words such as "natural," "meatless," and "organic" are in every grocery store. Vegetarianism is being promoted for better health and reduction of many chronic illnesses and conditions. The paradigm changed because of both an accumulation of data in the medical literature and social change, resulting in gradual removal of the blinders of bias.

The Politics of Environmental Health

Environmental health issues are percolating on every political agenda. Right-wing politicians purposely keep their heads down in order to avoid the ethically correct political decision to legislate reduction of pollution.

It goes against the grain of free enterprise and is not fiscally responsible — until you factor in the health costs. Left-wingers are looked upon as tree-hugging eco-terrorists who would like to dismantle the entire economic structure of the Western world in order to reduce pollution now. Meanwhile, when governmental decisions are made on your behalf, all the stakeholders are represented in that decision-making process, including both the chemical industry and the environmentalists. Or so it appears. The rising stakes of global warming and increasing evidence for the impact of pollution on disease raise the question of why Environment Canada recently eliminated 300 positions. The jobs lost included engineers, scientists, biologists, climatologists, and chemical analysts from across the country, working in such areas as pollution studies, water quality monitoring, and climate research. According to a government spokesperson, "While difficult, this decision will allow our government to continue to invest in clear air and a healthier environment for Canadians." Huh?

My limited understanding of our political system is that whoever is in power eventually loses power to the other side, after they screw up enough to make sufficient numbers of people so angry that they actually go out and vote against them. Depending on government to figure out how to protect the population from pollution, at the same time as it is promoting financial growth to ensure or even improve our present lifestyle, is at minimum extremely naive, perhaps even oxymoronic. And don't get me started on the American political system's track record on pollution, whether it is banning chemicals while producing them for export to the countries in the developing world or sending massive amounts of coal-burning air pollution into southern Ontario.

Children exposed to more air pollution perform worse on tests of cognitive functioning and have reduced working memory, impaired neurological function, and lower IQ scores. On a municipal level, the decision-makers might build new schools far away from major roadways, or refuse to license daycare centres that are too close. Maybe they could find or raise enough funds to improve the indoor air quality in older schools to enhance school performance.

Studies show that improvement of indoor air quality beyond the existing minimal standards increases office productivity. Here's a question: should businesses minimize ventilation to reduce energy costs and carbon emissions or maximize it to improve health and enhance the performance of their employees? Given that the biggest cost to the employer is employees, especially through absenteeism and poor work performance, the cost-benefit analysis would likely suggest that improved productivity is more cost-effective. This would work even better if the indoor air contamination were reduced too, starting with a no-scent policy, which doesn't cost anything. How cost-effective is that? These are incentives to change, even for your average Consumerian.

As a condition of hosting the 2008 Olympic Games, the Chinese government agreed to substantially (and temporarily) improve air quality in Beijing during the games and the subsequent Paralympics. A series of aggressive pollution-control measures was implemented that encompassed the entire Olympic and Paralympic Games. They limited the operation of industrial and commercial combustion facilities in Beijing and enforced alternate-day driving rules to remove approximately half the cars (about 1.5 million vehicles) from Beijing roads each day. Because of these changes, concentrations of particulate and gaseous pollutants decreased substantially; after the Paralympics they increased again, when the pollution control measures were relaxed.

The marked changes in air pollution before, during, and after the games provided a unique opportunity to investigate whether improving air quality could actually make a difference in health. Until the pollution controls were discontinued, there were reductions in biomarkers for clotting, inflammation, and systolic blood pressure in young, healthy subjects. There were also temporary reductions in pulmonary inflammation in children, and reduced risk for heart attack in taxi drivers.

Around the world other national or regional air pollution reductions have taken place, for various reasons such as governmental policy, national political realignment (for example, the reunification of Germany), employee strikes at industrial facilities, or large-scale sporting events. Every time pollution reductions occur, an associated beneficial public health effect has been observed, including reduced preterm deliveries, hospital admissions of children for respiratory disease and asthma, prevalence of bronchitis, and cardio-respiratory mortality rates.

Clearly it's time to change how we think. Waiting for the government to act in a timely manner is ludicrous. It's not just the politics. Asking the chemical producers and manufacturing industries to put human health before profit goes against the opinions of most CEOs and their shareholders. It's simply not going to happen.

So whom do you trust to advise you about the potential significance of environmental exposures to your health? Not the government, whose motivation is politically driven; not the manufacturing industry, whose bottom line is money; and hopefully not the mass media, which deliver information gathered by people who are trained as journalists, with limited education, if any, about the subject at hand. It's even worse with the internet, where absolutely anyone, without any credentials, can blog their own propaganda with apparent authority.

It looks as if we will need to depend on our health care practitioners. The theory is that they are not biased and are motivated and trained to provide advice gleaned from objective peer-reviewed, high-quality science to improve your health from an environmental perspective. Unfortunately, at present that's still just a theory. Recently a young medical resident showed wisdom beyond his years when he exclaimed, "I probably received five minutes of training in environmental medicine when I was in medical school. How can I have an opinion?"

The New Era of Environmental Medicine

In the early 1990s the Institute of Medicine was already advising doctors to be prepared to diagnose, prevent, and treat environmentally related conditions. Public trust in government and industry was declining and physicians were being looked upon by patients and community groups as reliable sources of information on environmental risks. In 1996, 24 percent of medical schools in the United States had no environmental content in their required curriculum. Those schools that did averaged only a total of seven hours of instruction, and 70 percent of the deans of those schools stated that there was minimal emphasis on environmental health. Environmental medicine was rated as an unimportant area of training by medical students and was described by physicians as the least important area in their practice.

Even now many doctors reveal that they are uninformed when questioned by their patients on possible environmental health effects. There is a reluctance among family doctors to widen their knowledge and practice of environmental medicine, because of their perception that the individual doctor–patient relationship should be dedicated mainly to treatment. As a result, submissions to present lectures to large numbers of physicians in medical education plenary sessions are frequently rejected. This in turn results in an inability among doctors to recognize the numerous times when it would be appropriate, or even necessary, to take an environmental exposure history.

I am reminded of a tragic case in which a middle-aged woman lived in a home with repeated water leaks in her basement whenever it rained. She had been mildly asthmatic for many years before moving into that house. Afterwards she developed such significant respiratory complaints that they could be controlled only with oral steroids. She was subsequently diagnosed with hypersensitivity pneumonitis, a progressive lung disease that eventually killed her. The cause of her disease was chronic mould exposure, which was not picked up by her physicians until a year later, because no one had thought to take an environmental exposure history.

The good news is that the Canadian College of Family Physicians has just inaugurated an accredited (Mainpro-C) two-day workshop on environmental medicine for practising physicians. Accumulation of Mainpro-C credits is necessary for family doctors who wish to earn or maintain their fellowship in the college. Together, my colleagues on the

Environmental Health Committee of the Ontario College of Family Physicians and I developed the workshop. But it's only a start. These workshops should be mandatory for all medical residents. Their basic concepts should be reviewed in plenary sessions in continuing medical education conferences, including those for all the appropriate specialties. And since all first-year medical students learn to take a history from their patients, teaching them how to take an environmental exposure history should be mandatory in every medical school.

First Do No Harm

We're both professionals. This is personal.

— Karl, in *Die Hard*

There is one condemnation of environmental physicians that remains to be addressed. This is in regard to the diagnosis of multiple chemical sensitivities (MCS). To me the most condescending and outrageous attack on environmental physicians was to blame us for our patients' illness because we supported their supposedly misguided attribution that chemical exposures were making them sick. The word used is *iatrogenic*, meaning "induced by the physician." Note the following quotes, describing patients seen by environmental physicians, from published and subsequently cited studies:

- ☐ If the patient does not discern his/her personal reality, it may be available from a clinical ecology centre, where patients have reported being diagnosed with a "chemically induced life-threatening illness" in an initial 5-min telephone evaluation by a receptionist.
- ☐ They are subjected to unnecessary harm and suffering inflicted by misguided or dishonest health care providers — the iatrogenic component.

☐ They have a cornucopia of pseudoscientific theories to draw from, with enough allusion to scientific studies to make their speculations alluring and seemingly plausible.

☐ The greatest challenge in treatment is to overcome the patient's disabling belief in a toxicogenic explanation for his or her symptoms.

The suggested treatment by those who continue to deny the biological basis for MCS is based on a psychiatric diagnosis; it includes deprogramming the patients by using desensitization. They describe an occasional successful case. Earlier I described the case of L.E., who was subjected to this treatment. Hers is an example of iatrogenic illness caused by a treatment proposed by deniers of MCS.

What do the patients have to say? In a survey of more than 900 patients with MCS, by looking at various treatments tried and comparing the likelihood of being helped versus being harmed, the following statistics were gleaned. The help/harm ratio was calculated as follows:

☐ chemical-free living space — 155:1 (most beneficial treatment)
☐ chemical avoidance — 119:1
☐ psychotherapy to help cope — 6:1
☐ psychotherapy for MCS cure — 1:1 (no help, but no harm)
☐ anti-anxiety/antidepressant medications — 0.3:1 (made it worse).

But, hey, what do the patients know?

The End

Choose your paradigms with an open mind and a clear perspective. If you want to address your journey along the oxidative stress continuum, any reduction of environmental exposures will have to be self-directed.

Since you are likely going to have to do it on your own, gather your information and make your decisions with wisdom. I hope that this book has provided you with some of that information and will motivate you to change your personal environment and lifestyle accordingly, to the best of your ability, to improve the quality of your life. Don't be oxidatively stressed out; stop the slide along the continuum. Take a multidisciplinary, (w)holistic systems medicine approach to better health and healthier aging. And take care of your children.

Listen to my grandmother — there are no more excuses. That should be your new paradigm.

GLOSSARY

Allostasis the process of achieving *homeostasis* or balance; adaptation.

Allostatic load the long-term effect on the body caused by repeated efforts to adapt.

Amygdala the part of the *limbic system* responsible for memory and emotional processing. It is linked to both fear and pleasure and is anatomically connected to *olfaction*.

Anaerobic threshold the point at which the oxygen supply becomes insufficient to maintain energy production.

Analgesic a substance that relieves pain.

Anaphylaxis a rapidly progressing systemic allergic reaction that can potentially result in complete airway obstruction, shock, and death.

Ankylosing spondylitis chronic inflammation of the spine and sacroiliac joints.

Antibody a specialized immune protein produced because of the introduction of an *antigen* into the body, able to recognize and combine with the very antigen that triggered its production.

Antigen any substance that invokes a specific immune response, such as the production or release of *antibodies*.

Antipyretic a substance that reduces fever.

Atherosclerosis progressive thickening and hardening of the walls of arteries as a result of deposits of fats and *cholesterol* (plaque), which can restrict blood flow.

Autoantibody an *antibody* that reacts with one's own cells, proteins, or tissues.

Autoimmune response an immune system reaction directed against the body's own cells or tissues.

Autonomic nervous system the part of the nervous system that regulates involuntary functions of the body, such as heart rate and digestion.

Basophil an immune cell involved in inflammation and allergies that releases *histamine*.

Biogenesis reproduction of living organisms.

Biopsychosocial approach an approach in medicine that considers the complex interactions of biology, the emotions, and social conditions.

Bisphenol A (BPA) an organic compound used to make high-performance polycarbonate plastic and epoxy resins found in many commonly used products.

BMI body mass index, a measurement of body fat calculated from height and weight.

Capsaicin the component of hot peppers that causes the sensation of burning.

CFS chronic fatigue syndrome.

Cholesterol fat produced by the liver that is the precursor of bile acids and steroid *hormones* and which builds and maintains cell membranes.

Cilia tiny, hair-like processes that extend from a cell's surface.

Circadian rhythm the daily rhythmic cycle, based on 24-hour intervals, which is exhibited by many organisms.

Co-morbidity the presence of two or more independent medical conditions.

Control group a group of people used as a standard of comparison in research studies.

COPD chronic obstructive pulmonary (lung) disease.

Criteria air pollutants common air pollutants for which the *EPA* has set permissible limits, using criteria based on human health and/or environmental concerns.

Cytokine a small protein messenger released by immune system cells that promotes inflammation and communicates with the brain.

DNA deoxyribonucleic acid, the main constituent of chromosomes that carry our genetic information.

DOHaD developmental origins of health and disease.

Dyslipidemia elevation of "bad" *cholesterol* (*LDL*) and/or *triglycerides*, and/or reduction of "good" cholesterol (*HDL*).

Endoplasmic reticulum cellular *organelles* that synthesize, modify, fold, and transport proteins.

Eosinophilic esophagitis an allergic inflammation of the esophagus.

EPA Environmental Protection Agency, U.S. federal government agency whose mission is to protect human health and the environment by creating and enforcing regulations based on laws passed by Congress.

Epidemiology the study of the patterns of disease in a population.

Epigenetics the process that alters gene activity and expression without actually changing the *DNA*.

Epigenome *epigenetic* control of genes.

Etiology the cause of a disease or condition.

Exposome a measure of all the exposures of an individual from conception to death and how those exposures relate to health, considering everything that is not due to the *genome*.

Flora the population of *microbes* that inhabit the outside and inside surfaces of humans.

Free radical an unstable molecule with an unpaired electron, capable of destabilizing neighbouring molecules by donating that electron or else stealing one from them.

Functional brain scan a method of scanning the human brain to study the activity in various parts.

Genome the entire genetic information of an organism.

GERD gastroesophageal reflux disease, a disorder that causes stomach acids to back up into the esophagus, its most common symptom being heartburn.

Gluten a protein found in wheat, barley, and rye.

Half-life the time required for half the amount of a chemical to be broken down or eliminated from the body.

HDL high-density lipoprotein; *cholesterol* wrapped in a large amount of protein that is also known as "good cholesterol."

Hippocampus the part of the *limbic system* that helps regulate emotion, learning, and memory.

Histamine a chemical mediator released by the immune cells that causes dilation of blood vessels, usually released in allergic reactions.

Homeostasis balance in the *metabolism*.

Hormone a chemical substance produced in one part of the body that travels through the bloodstream to control and regulate the function of other cells or organs.

HPA *hypothalamus*–pituitary–adrenal axis, the pathway of the stress response from the brain to the adrenal glands.

Hypervigilance abnormally increased arousal and an abnormal awareness of environmental stimuli.

Hypothalamus the region of the brain that coordinates both the *autonomic nervous system* and the activity of the pituitary gland.

IgE immunoglobulin E, the type of *antibody* involved in allergic reactions.

IgG the most predominant type of *antibody*, formed in response to infecting agents and other foreign substances.

Immune-mediated disease a disease caused by the immune system.

Incidence the frequency or rate at which a certain event occurs; the number of new cases of a specific disease that occurs during a certain period in a specific population.

Iritis inflammation of the iris of the eye.

LDL low-density lipoprotein; *cholesterol* wrapped in a minimal amount of protein that is also known as "bad cholesterol."

Limbic system the group of structures in the brain responsible for survival and adaptation to the environment. It is involved in primitive emotions such as fear and anger, motivation, and emotional associations with memories.

Lipids fats carried in the bloodstream, made up mostly of *cholesterol* and *triglycerides*.

Mast cell an immune cell commonly involved in allergic reactions that produces *histamine* and *cytokines*.

MCS multiple chemical sensitivities.

ME myalgic encephalomyelitis, also known as chronic fatigue syndrome (ME/CFS).

Metabolism the biochemical processes that maintain life.

Metabolic syndrome a combination of insulin resistance, obesity, high blood pressure, and *dyslipidemia*.

Microbes minute life forms such as bacteria, viruses, or parasites.

Microbial flora a population of *microbes*.

Microbiome the gene pool of all the *microbes* living on or in humans.

Microbiota the collection of *microbes* that live on and inside humans.

Microflora bacteria and other microorganisms.

Mitochondria the cellular *organelles* that produce energy (singular: mitochondrion).

Morbidity a condition or state of disease; the *incidence* or *prevalence* of a disease in a population.

Motility the ability to move spontaneously and actively.

Multi-morbidity the co-occurrence of two or more chronic conditions.

Mutualism when two species contribute to each other's success and survival.

Neuron a nerve cell.

Neurotransmitter a chemical messenger released by a nerve cell to provoke a response in a neighbouring cell.

Nucleus the cellular *organelle* that contains the *DNA*.

Olfaction the sense of smell.

Organelle a component of a cell with a specific function.

Organic a molecule that contains carbon; food produced, processed, and transported without the use of commercial chemicals such as fertilizers, pesticides, or synthetic substances that enhance colour or flavour.

Oxidant a molecule capable of stealing an electron from a neighbouring molecule, causing damage to its structure.

Oxidation the act of stealing an electron from another molecule.

Oxidative stress an imbalance between the level of *oxidants* in an organism and its ability to detoxify them.

Particulate matter small, discrete masses of solid or liquid matter that remain suspended in the air for long periods of time.

Pollutant a substance that contaminates an environment, may have undesirable effects, and is potentially harmful to humans.

POP persistent organic pollutant, a *pollutant* that degrades extremely slowly.

Precautionary principle an ethic dictating that when human activities might lead to morally unacceptable harm that is scientifically plausible but uncertain, actions should be taken to avoid or diminish that harm.

Prevalence the percentage of a population that has a particular disease or condition at a given time.

Psoriasis a chronic *autoimmune* disease of the skin.

Psychoneuroimmunology the field of medicine that deals with the bidirectional influences and actions between the brain and the immune system.

Receptor a structure on the surface of a cell that selectively receives and binds a specific substance in order to receive a message and initiate a response.

SBS sick building syndrome.

Scleroderma an *autoimmune* disease of the connective tissue of the skin.

Semi-volatile a substance that evaporates slowly at normal temperatures.

Sensitization the process of becoming susceptible to a stimulus that previously had no effect or significance.

SIBO small intestine bacterial overgrowth.

Sleep apnea a chronic medical condition that causes repeated cessation of breathing during sleep.

Somatization the unconscious process by which psychological distress is expressed as bodily symptoms.

Sublingal challenge test performed by placing an extract of a substance such as a food under the tongue in an attempt to provoke a reaction that duplicates the individual's symptoms.

SVOC semi-volatile organic compounds, which tend to vaporize slowly at room temperature and less than *VOCs*.

Synapse the space or junction where a *neuron* can communicate with a neighbouring cell.

Terpene a naturally derived *organic* chemical that comes from the essential oils of plants.

Tight junction a space between cells where they are tightly held together to provide a barrier.

Triglyceride a type of *lipid* that makes up most of the fat in the body, synthesized from fats and oils.

TRPV1 receptor transient *receptor* potential cation channel, subfamily V, member 1. Sensitive to *capsaicin*, it is found in many areas of the body and functions as a general sensor of noxious stimuli, responsible for *sensitization* to chemicals.

TVOC total amount of *volatile organic compounds*.

VOC volatile organic compound; any compound of carbon — excluding carbon monoxide and carbon dioxide — that can evaporate at normal air temperatures and pressure.

Volatile evaporates readily at normal temperatures.

Xenobiotics man-made chemical substances that are foreign to an organism, including drugs and *pollutants*.

FURTHER READING

Chapter 3: Everyone's Got an Opinion

Craig, W.J. "Position of the American Dietetic Association: Vegetarian Diets." *Journal of the American Dietetic Association* 109, no. 7 (2009): 1266–82.

Lindbloom, E.J. "Long-Term Benefits of a Vegetarian Diet." *American Family Physician* 79, no. 7 (2009): 541–42.

Thomson, G.M. *Report of the Ad Hoc Committee on Environmental Hypersensitivity Disorders.* Toronto: Ontario Ministry of Health, August 1985.

Chapter 4: Outdoor Air

Boothe, V.L. "Potential Health Effects Associated with Residential Proximity to Freeways and Primary Roads: Review of Scientific Literature, 1999–2006." *Journal of Environmental Health* 70, no. 8 (2008): 33–41.

Brook, R.D. "Particulate Matter, Air Pollution and Cardiovascular Disease: An Update to the Scientific Statement from the American Heart Association." *Circulation* 121 (2010): 2331–78.

Browner, C. *Environmental Health Threats to Children*. EPA 175-F-96-110. Washington, DC: U.S. Environmental Protection Agency, 1996.

Cohen, A.J. "The Global Burden of Disease Due to Outdoor Air Pollution." *Journal of Toxicology and Environmental Health* A. 68, no. 13/14 (2005): 1301–7.

Crawford, E. *Smog and Population Health*. PRB 05-101E. Ottawa: Parliamentary Information and Research Service, March 28, 2006.

Ostro, B. *Outdoor Pollution: Assessing the Environmental Burden of Disease at National and Local Levels*. Environmental Burden of Disease Series 5. Geneva: World Health Organization, 2004.

World Health Organization. "Health Aspects of Air Pollution with Particulate Matter, Ozone and Nitrogen Dioxide." Report of WHO working group, Bonn, Germany, January 13–15, 2003. http://www.euro.who.int/_data/assets/pdf_file/0005/112199/E79097.pdf (accessed July 18, 2012).

Chapter 5: The Body Burden

Centers for Disease Control and Prevention. *Fourth National Report on Human Exposure to Environmental Chemicals*. Atlanta, GA: CDC, 2009.

Health Canada. *Report on Human Biomonitoring of Environmental Chemicals in Canada, 2010*. http://www.hc-sc.gc.ca/ewh-semt/alt_formats/hecs-sesc/pdf/pubs/contaminants/chms-ecms/report-rapport-eng.pdf (accessed July 11, 2011).

U.S. Environmental Protection Agency. *EPA National Human Adipose Tissue Survey* (1979–83). http://cfpub.epa.gov/ncea/cfm/recordisplay.cfm?deid=55204 (accessed July 18, 2012).

Chapter 6: Indoor Air

Canadian Centre for Occupational Health and Safety. "Scent-Free Policy for the Workplace." http://www.ccohs.ca/oshanswers/hsprograms/scent_free.html (accessed July 18, 2012).

Caress, S.M. "Prevalence of Fragrance Sensitivity in the American Population." *Journal of Environmental Health* 71, no. 7 (2009): 46–50.

European Commission. *European Collaborative Action: Indoor Air Quality and Its Impact on Man*. Total Volatile Organic Compounds (TVOC) in Indoor Air Quality. Investigations, report 19. Luxembourg: Office for Official Publications of the European Communities, 1997.

Lax, M.B. "Patients with Multiple Chemical Sensitivities in an Occupational Health Clinic: Presentation and Follow-up." *Archives of Environmental Health* 50 (1995): 425–31.

Levin, H. *National Programs to Assess IEQ Effects of Building Materials and Products*. Washington, DC: EPA, September 17, 2010. http://www.epa.gov/iaq/pdfs/hal_levin_paper.pdf (accessed July 18, 2012).

Logue, J.M. "Hazard Assessment of Chemical Air Contaminants Measured in Residences." *Indoor Air* 21 (2011): 92–109.

Mitchell, C.S. "Current State of the Science: Health Effects and Indoor Environmental Quality." *Environmental Health Perspectives* 115, no. 6 (2007): 958–64.

Steinemann, A.C. "Fragranced Consumer Products and Undisclosed Ingredients." *Environmental Impact Assessment Review* 29 (2009): 32–38.

Steinemann, A.C. "Fragranced Consumer Products: Chemicals Emitted, Ingredients Unlisted." *Environmental Impact Assessment Review* 31, no. 3 (2011): 328–33.

Weschler, C.J. "Chemistry in Indoor Environments: 20 Years of Research." *Indoor Air* 21 (2011): 205–18.

Chapter 7: How Our Bodies Cope

Bratic, I. "Mitochondrial Energy Metabolism and Ageing." *Biochimica et Biophysica Acta* 1797, no. 6/7 (2010): 961–67.

Hong, Y.C. "Community Level Exposure to Chemicals and Oxidative Stress in Adult Population." *Toxicology Letters* 184 (2009): 139–44.

Loeb, L.A. "The Mitochondrial Theory of Aging and Its Relationship to Reactive Oxygen Species Damage and Somatic mtDNA Mutations." *Proceedings of the National Academy of Sciences* 102, no. 52 (2005): 18769–70.

Lu, C.Y. "Oxidative DNA Damage Estimated by Urinary 8-hydroxydeoxyguanosine and Indoor Air Pollution among Non-smoking Office Employees." *Environmental Research* 103, no. 3 (2007): 331–37.

"Oxidative Stress Associated with Indoor Air Pollution and Sick Building Syndrome–Related Symptoms among Office Workers in Taiwan." *Inhalation Toxicology* 19 (2007): 57–65.

Chapter 8: MCS Exists

Elberling, J. "The Capsaicin Cough Reflex in Eczema Patients with Respiratory Symptoms Elicited by Perfume." *Contact Dermatitis* 54, no. 3 (2006): 158–64.

Gilbert, M.E. "Does the Kindling Model of Epilepsy Contribute to Our Understanding of Multiple Chemical Sensitivity?" *Annals of the New York Academy of Sciences* 933 (2001): 68–91.

Heuser, G. "Deep Subcortical (Including Limbic) Hypermetabolism in Patients with Chemical Intolerance: Human PET Studies." *Annals of the New York Academy of Sciences* 933 (2001): 319–22.

Holst, H. "The Capsaicin Cough Reflex in Patients with Symptoms Elicited by Odorous Chemicals." *International Journal of Hygiene and Environmental Health* 213, no. 1 (2010): 66–71.

Millqvist, E. "Changes in Levels of Nerve Growth Factor in Nasal Secretions after Capsaicin Inhalation in Patients with Airway Symptoms from Scents and Chemicals." *Environmental Health Perspectives* 113, no. 7 (2005): 849–52.

Millqvist, E. "Relationship of Airway Symptoms from Chemicals to Capsaicin Cough Sensitivity in Atopic Subjects." *Clinical and Experimental Allergy* 34, no. 4 (2004): 619–23.

Orriols, R. "Brain Dysfunction in Multiple Chemical Sensitivity." *Journal of the Neurological Sciences* 287, no. 1/2 (2009): 72–78.

Terneston-Hasseus, E. "Increased Capsaicin Cough Sensitivity in Patients with Multiple Chemical Sensitivity." *Journal of Occupational and Environmental Medicine* 44, no. 11 (2002): 1012–17.

Chapter 9: Connecting the Dots

Barsky, A.J. "Functional Somatic Syndromes." *Annals of Internal Medicine* 130, no. 11 (1999): 910–21.

Chapter 10: Sick and Tired

Andersen, S.L. "Preliminary Evidence for Sensitive Periods in the Effect of Childhood Sexual Abuse on Regional Brain Development." *Journal of Neuropsychiatry and Clinical Neurosciences* 20 (2008): 292–301.

Blankstein, U. "Altered Brain Structure in Irritable Bowel Syndrome: Potential Contributions of Pre-existing and Disease-Driven Factors." *Gastroenterology* 138, no. 5 (2010): 1783–89.

Dantzer, R. "Twenty Years of Research on Cytokine-Induced Sickness Behavior." *Brain, Behavior and Immunity* 21, no. 2 (2007): 153–60.

Dantzer. R., J.D. O'Connor, G.G. Freund, et al. "From Inflammation to Sickness and Depression: When the Immune System Subjugates the Brain." *Nature Reviews Neuroscience* 9 (2008): 46–56.

Ghazan-Shahi, S. "Should Rheumatologists Retain Ownership of Fibromyalgia? A Survey of Ontario Rheumatologists." *Clinical Rheumatology* 31, no. 8 (2012): 1177–81.

Griffith, J.P. "A Systematic Review of Chronic Fatigue Syndrome: Don't Assume It's Depression." *Primary Care Companion to the Journal of Clinical Psychiatry* 10 (2008): 120–28.

Jason, L.A. "Chronic Fatigue Syndrome, Fibromyalgia, and Multiple Chemical Sensitivities in a Community-Based Sample of Persons with Chronic Fatigue Syndrome–Like Symptoms." *Psychosomatic Medicine* 62, no. 5 (2000): 655–63.

Miller, G.E. "Psychological Stress in Childhood and Susceptibility to the Chronic Diseases of Aging: Moving Toward a Model of Behavioral and Biological Mechanisms." *Psychological Bulletin* 137, no. 6 (2011): 959–97.

Petersen, D.L. "Central Amplification and Fibromyalgia: Disorder of Pain Processing." *Journal of Neuroscience Research* 89, no. 1 (2011): 29–34.

Rainville, P. "Representation of Acute and Persistent Pain in the Human CNS: Potential Implications for Chemical Intolerance." *Annals of the New York Academy of Sciences* 933 (2001): 130–41.

Szyszkowicz, M. "Air Pollution and Daily Emergency Department Visits for Depression." *International Journal of Occupational Medicine and Environmental Health* 22, no. 4 (2009): 355–62.

Tran, M.T. "Multiple Chemical Sensitivity: On the Scent of Central Sensitization." *International Journal of Hygiene and Environmental Health* 216, no. 2 (2013): 202–10.

Ursin, H. "Sensitization, Subjective Health Complaints, and Sustained Arousal." *Annals of the New York Academy of Sciences* 933 (2001): 119–29.

Wegman, H.L. "A Meta-analytic Review of the Effects of Childhood Abuse on Medical Outcomes in Adulthood." *Psychosomatic Medicine* 71, no. 8 (2009): 805–12.

Wolfe, F. "The American College of Rheumatology Preliminary Diagnostic Criteria for Fibromyalgia and Measurement of Symptom Severity." *Arthritis Care and Research* 62, no. 5 (2010): 600–610.

Chapter 11: More Dots to Connect

Backhed, F. "The Gut Microbiota as an Environmental Factor that Regulates Fat Storage." *Proceedings of the National Academy of Sciences of the United States* 101 (2004): 15718–23.

Bager, P. "Caesarean Section and Offspring's Risk of Inflammatory Bowel Disease: A National Cohort Study." *Inflammatory Bowel Diseases* 18, no. 5 (2012): 857–62.

"Mode of Delivery and Risk of Allergic Rhinitis and Asthma." *Journal of Allergy and Clinical Immunology* 111 (2003): 51–56.

Cardwell, C.R. "Caesarean Section Is Associated with an Increased Risk of Childhood-Onset Type 1 Diabetes Mellitus: A Meta-analysis of Observational Studies." *Diabetologia* 51 (2008): 726–35.

Huh, S.Y. "Delivery by Caesarean Section and Risk of Obesity in Preschool Age Children: A Prospective Cohort Study." *Archives of Disease in Childhood* 97, no. 7 (2012): 610–16.

Turnbaugh, P.J. "The Human Microbiome Project." *Nature* 449 (2007): 804–10.

Chapter 13: Obesity

Adam, C. "Stress, Eating and the Reward System." *Physiology and Behavior* 91, no. 4 (2007): 449–58.

Baillie-Hamilton, P.F. "Chemical Toxins: A Hypothesis to Explain the Global Obesity Epidemic." *Journal of Alternative and Complementary Medicine* 8 (2002): 185–92.

Birnbaum, L.S. "Environmental Chemicals: Evaluating Low-Dose Effects." *Environmental Health Perspectives* 120, no. 4 (2012): A143–44.

Bruce, A.S. "Obese Children Show Hyperactivation to Food Pictures in Brain Networks Linked to Motivation, Reward and Cognitive Control." *International Journal of Obesity* 34, no. 10 (2010): 1494–500.

Martin, L.E. "Neural Mechanisms Associated with Food Motivation in Obese and Healthy Weight Adults." *Obesity* 18, no. 2 (2010): 254–60.

Newbold, R.R. "Impact of Environmental Endocrine Disrupting Chemicals on the Development of Obesity." *Hormones* 9, no. 3 (2010): 206–17.

Obesity: Preventing and Managing the Global Epidemic. Report of a WHO Consultation. Report 894. Geneva: World Health Organization, 2000. http://www.who.int/nutrition/publications/obesity/WHO_TRS_894/en/index.html (accessed July 18, 2012).

Ogden, C.L. "Prevalence of High Body Mass Index in U.S. Children and Adolescents, 2007–2008." *Journal of the American Medical Association* 303 (2010): 242–49.

Pou, K.M. "Visceral and Subcutaneous Adipose Tissue Volumes Are Cross-Sectionally Related to Markers of Inflammation and Oxidative Stress: The Framingham Heart Study." *Circulation* 116 (2007): 1234–41.

Rundle, A. "Association of Childhood Obesity with Maternal Exposure to Ambient Air Polycyclic Aromatic Hydrocarbons During Pregnancy." *American Journal of Epidemiology* 175, no. 11 (2012): 1163–72.

Teachman, B.A. "Demonstrations of Implicit Anti-fat Bias: The Impact of Providing Causal Information and Evoking Empathy." *Journal of Health Psychology* 22 (2003): 68–78.

World Health Organization. "Executive Summary." *Global Assessment of the State-of-the-Science of Endocrine Disruptors.* Geneva: WHO International Programme on Chemical Safety, 2003. http://www.who.int/ipcs/publications/en/ch1.pdf (accessed July 18, 2012).

Chapter 14: Reductionism and Systems Biology

Ahn, A.C. "The Clinical Application of a Systems Approach." *PLoS Medicine* 3, no. 7 (2006): e209.

Andreazza, A.C. "Oxidative Stress Markers in Bipolar Disorder: A Meta-analysis." *Journal of Affective Disorders* 111, no. 2/3 (2008): 135–44.

Kitano, H. "Systems Biology: A Brief Overview." *Science* 295 (2002): 1662–64.

Marazziti, D. "Mitochondrial Alterations and Neuropsychiatric Disorders." *Current Medicinal Chemistry* 18, no. 30 (2011): 4715–21.

Seeman, T.E. "Price of Adaptation: Allostatic Load and Its Health Consequences." *Archives of Internal Medicine* 157 (1997): 2259–68.

Strange, K. "The End of 'Naïve Reductionism': Rise of Systems Biology or Renaissance of Physiology?" *American Journal of Physiology Cell Physiology* 288 (2005): C968–74.

Chapter 15: The Oxidative Stress Continuum

Almgren, T. "Stroke and Coronary Heart Disease in Treated Hypertension: A Prospective Cohort Study over Three Decades." *Journal of Internal Medicine* 257, no. 6 (2005): 496–502.

Altindag, O. "Total Antioxidant Capacity and the Severity of the Pain in Patients with Fibromyalgia." *Redox Report* 11, no. 3 (2006): 131–35.

Andersson, O.K. "Survival in Treated Hypertension: Follow up Study after Two Decades." *BMJ* 317, no. 7152 (1998): 167–71.

Behan, W.M.H. "Mitochondrial Abnormalities in the Postviral Fatigue Syndrome." *Acta Neuropathologica* 83 (1991): 61–65.

Centers for Disease Control and Prevention. "About Heart Disease & Stroke: Consequences & Costs." *Million Hearts*. http://millionhearts.hhs.gov/abouthds/costconsequences. html (accessed December 12, 2012).

Eriksson, U.K. "Asthma, Eczema, Rhinitis and the Risk for Dementia." *Dementia and Geriatric Cognitive Disorders* 25, no. 2 (2008): 148–56.

Gasana, J. "Motor Vehicle Air Pollution and Asthma in Children: A Meta-analysis." *Environmental Research* 117 (2012): 36–45.

Hardeland, R. "Circadian Rhythms, Oxidative Stress, and Antioxidative Defense Mechanisms." *Chronobiology International* 20, no. 6 (2003): 921–62.

Iqbal, R. "Pathophysiology and Antioxidant Status of Patients with Fibromyalgia." *Rheumatology International* 31, no. 2 (February 2011): 149–52.

Jammes, Y. "Chronic Fatigue Syndrome: Assessment of Increased Oxidative Stress and Altered Muscle Excitability in Response to Incremental Exercise." *Journal of Internal Medicine* 257 (2005): 299–310.

Kennedy, G. "Oxidative Stress Levels Are Raised in Chronic Fatigue Syndrome and Are Associated with Clinical Symptoms." *Free Radical Biology and Medicine* 39, no. 5 (2005): 584–89.

Kim, J. "Relation Between Common Allergic Symptoms and Coronary Heart Disease among NHANES III Participants." *American Journal of Cardiology* 106, no. 7 (2010): 984–87.

Lavergne, R. "Functional Impairment in Chronic Fatigue Syndrome, Fibromyalgia and Multiple Chemical Sensitivity." *Canadian Family Physician* 56 (2010): e57–65.

Maes, M. "A Review on the Oxidative and Nitrosative stress (O&NS) Pathways in Major Depression and Their Possible Contribution to the (Neuro)degenerative Processes in that Illness." *Progress in Neuro-Psychopharmacology and Biological Psychiatry* 35, no. 3 (2011): 676–92.

Maheswaran, R. "Impact of Outdoor Air Pollution on Survival after Stroke." *Stroke* 41 (2010): 869–77.

Oberdorster, G. "Translocation of Inhaled Ultrafine Particles to the Brain." *Inhalation Toxicology* 16, no. 6/7 (2004): 437–45.

Ontario Ministry of Health and Long-Term Care. Preventing and Managing Chronic Disease: Ontario's Framework. May 2007. http://www.health.gov.on.ca/en/pro/programs/cdpm/pdf/framework_full.pdf (accessed July 11, 2013).

Public Health Agency of Canada. *Tracking Heart Disease and Stroke in Canada*. June 2009. http://www.phac-aspc.gc.ca/publicat/2009/cvd-avc/index-eng.php (accessed August 31, 2012).

Takenoue, Y. "The Influence of Outdoor NO2 Exposure on Asthma in Childhood: A Meta-analysis." *Pediatrics International* 54, no. 6 (2012): 762–69.

Torresani, C. "Chronic Urticaria Is Usually Associated with Fibromyalgia Syndrome." *Acta Dermato-Venereologica* 89, no. 4 (2009): 389–92.

United States Department of Health and Human Services. *Multiple Chronic Conditions: A Strategic Framework. Optimum Health and Quality of Life for Individuals with Multiple Chronic Conditions*. Washington, DC: HHS, December 2010. http://www.hhs.gov/ash/initiatives/mcc/mcc_framework.pdf (accessed July 18, 2012).

Van der Vliet, A. "Effect of Oxidative Stress on Receptors and Signal Transmission." *Chemico-Biological Interactions* 85, no. 2/3 (1992): 95–116.

Chapter 16: Women and Children First

Bierman, A.S., ed. *Project for an Ontario Women's Health Evidence-Based Report*, vol. 2. Toronto: POWER Study, 2010–12.

Boyle, C.A. "Trends in the Prevalence of Developmental Disabilities in U.S. Children, 1997–2008." *Pediatrics* 127, no. 6 (2011): 1034–42.

Centers for Disease Control and Prevention. "Prevalence of Autism Spectrum Disorders: Autism and Developmental Disabilities Monitoring Network, United States 2006." *Morbidity and Mortality Weekly Report Surveillance Summaries* 58, no. 10 (2009): 1–20.

Fowler, R.A. "Sex- and Age-Based Differences in the Delivery and Outcomes of Critical Care." *Canadian Medical Association Journal* 177 (2007): 1513–19.

Grandjean, P. "Developmental Neurotoxicity of Industrial Chemicals: A Silent Pandemic." *Lancet* 368 (2006): 2167–78.

Institute of Medicine Immunization Safety Review Committee, Board of Health Promotion and Disease Prevention. *Immunization Safety Review: Vaccines and Autism.* Washington, DC: National Academy Press, 2004.

Kalliomaki, M. "Early Differences in Fecal Microbiota Composition in Children May Predict Overweight." *American Journal of Clinical Nutrition* 87 (2008): 534–38.

Landrigan, P.J. "What Causes Autism? Exploring the Environmental Contribution." *Current Opinion in Pediatrics* 22 (2010): 219–25.

Narayan, K.M. "Lifetime Risk for Diabetes Mellitus in the United States." *Journal of the American Medical Association* 290, no. 14 (2003): 1884–90.

Perera, F.P. "Effect of Prenatal Exposure to Airborne Polycyclic Aromatic Hydrocarbons on Neurodevelopment in the First 3 Years of Life among Inner-City Children." *Environmental Health Perspectives* 114, no. 8 (2006): 1287–92.

Thavagnanam, S. "A Meta-analysis of the Association Between Caesarean Section and Childhood Asthma." *Clinical and Experimental Allergy* 38 (2008): 629–33.

Tran, C. "Gender Differences in Adverse Drug Reactions." *Journal of Clinical Pharmacology* 38 (1998): 1003–9.

United States Environmental Protection Agency, Office of Pollution Prevention and Toxic Substances. *Chemical Hazard Data Availability Study: What Do We Really Know about the Safety of High Production Volume Chemicals?* Washington, DC: EPA, 1998.

http://www.epa.gov/hpv/pubs/general/hazchem.pdf (accessed August 31, 2012).

Verbeeten, K.C. "Association Between Childhood Obesity and Subsequent Type 1 Diabetes: A Systematic Review and Meta-analysis." *Diabetic Medicine* 28 (2011):10–18.

Volk, H.E. "Residential Proximity to Freeways and Autism in the CHARGE Study." *Environmental Health Perspectives* 119, no. 6 (2011): 873–77.

Windham, G.C. "Autism Spectrum Disorders in Relation to Distribution of Hazardous Air Pollutants in the San Francisco Bay Area." *Environmental Health Perspectives* 114, no. 9 (2006): 1438–44.

Chapter 17: The Nine-Point Plan

Bo, H. "Redefining the Role of Mitochondria in Exercise: A Dynamic Remodeling." *Annals of the New York Academy of Sciences* 1201 (2010): 121–28.

Canadian Society for Exercise Physiology. *Canadian Physical Activity and Sedentary Behaviour Guidelines.* http://www.csep.ca/english/view.asp?x=804 (accessed April 9, 2012).

Chevrier, J. "Body Weight Loss Increases Plasma and Adipose Tissue Concentrations of Potentially Toxic Pollutants in Obese Individuals." *International Journal of Obesity* 24 (2000): 1272–78.

Dewell, A. "A Very-Low-Fat Vegan Diet Increases Intake of Protective Dietary Factors and Decreases Intake of Pathogenic Dietary Factors." *Journal of the American Dietetic Association* 108, no. 2 (2008): 347–56.

Genuis, S.J. "Blood, Urine, and Sweat (BUS) Study: Monitoring and Elimination of Bioaccumulated Toxic Elements." *Archives of Environmental Contamination and Toxicology* 61, no. 2 (2011): 344–57.

Hue, O. "Increased Plasma Levels of Toxic Pollutants Accompanying Weight Loss Induced by Hypocaloric Diet or by Bariatric Surgery." *Obesity Surgery* 16, no. 9 (2006): 1145–54.

Jones, D.E. "Loss of Capacity to Recover from Acidosis on Repeat Exercise in Chronic Fatigue Syndrome: A Case-Control Study." *European Journal of Clinical Investigation* 42, no. 2 (2012): 186–94.

Ohori, T. "Effect of Repeated Sauna Treatment on Exercise Tolerance and Endothelial Function in Patients with Chronic Heart Failure." *American Journal of Cardiology* 109, no. 1 (2012): 100–104.

Ostergaard, J.N. "Combined Effects of Weight Loss and Physical Activity on All-Cause Mortality of Overweight Men and Women." *International Journal of Obesity* 34, no. 4 (2010): 760–69.

Pilch, W. "Changes in the Lipid Profile of Blood Serum in Women Taking Sauna Baths of Various Duration." *International Journal of Occupational Medicine and Environmental Health* 23, no. 2 (2010): 167–74.

Chapter 23: The Politics of Medicine

Bakó-Biró, Z. "Effects of Pollution from Personal Computers on Perceived Air Quality, SBS Symptoms and Productivity in Offices." *Indoor Air* 14 (2004): 178–87.

Canadian Centre for Occupational Health and Safety. "Scent-Free Policy for the Workplace." *Health & Safety Programs.* 2010. http://www.ccohs.ca/oshanswers/hsprograms/scent_free.html (accessed August 31, 2012).

Canadian Lung Association. "Policy for Developing a Scent-Free Workplace." http://www.lung.ca/_resources/DevelopingaScentfreePolicyforaWorkplace.pdf (accessed August 31, 2012).

Centers for Disease Control and Prevention. *Indoor Environmental Quality.* http://www.cdc.gov/niosh/topics/indoorenv/ (accessed July 11, 2013).

Freire, C. "Association of Traffic-Related Air Pollution with Cognitive Development in Children." *Journal of Epidemiology and Community Health* 64, no. 3 (2010): 223.

Parker, J.D. "Preterm Birth after the Utah Valley Steel Mill Closure: A Natural Experiment." *Epidemiology* 19, no. 6 (2008): 820–23.

Sears, M. *The Medical Perspective on Environmental Sensitivities*. Ottawa: Canadian Human Rights Commission, 2007. http://www.chrc-ccdp.ca/sites/default/files/envsensitivity_en_1.pdf (accessed July 11, 2013).

Sunyer, J. "The Neurological Effects of Air Pollution in Children." *European Respiratory Journal* 32, no. 3 (2008): 535–37.

Wargocki, P. "The Effects of Outdoor Air Supply Rate and Supply Air Filter Condition in Classrooms on the Performance of Schoolwork by Children." *HVAC&R Research* 13, no. 2 (2011): 165–91.

INDEX